Staffordshire Library and Information Services
Please return or renew by the last date shown

If not required by other readers, this item may be renewed in person, by post or telephone, online or by email.
To renew, either the book or ticket are required.

24 Hour Renewal Line
0845 33 00 740

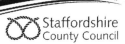
Staffordshire
County Council

M·U·D·R·A·S

YOGA
in your
HANDS

GERTRUD HIRSCHI

CORONET

This edition first published in Great Britain in 2016 by Coronet
An imprint of Hodder & Stoughton
An Hachette UK company

1

Copyright © Gertrud Hirschi 2000

The right of Gertrud Hirschi to be identified as the Author of the Work
has been asserted by her in accordance with the Copyright,
Designs and Patents Act 1988.

A CIP catalogue record for this title is available from the British Library

Paperback ISBN: 978 1 473 63213 4
Ebook ISBN: 978 1 473 63214 1

Printed and bound by Clays Ltd, St Ives plc

Hodder & Stoughton policy is to use papers that are natural, renewable
and recyclable products and made from wood grown in sustainable forests.
The logging and manufacturing processes are expected to conform to
the environmental regulations of the country of origin.

Hodder & Stoughton Ltd
Carmelite House
50 Victoria Embankment
London EC4Y 0DZ

www.hodder.co.uk

CONTENTS

Part One
EXPLORING THE MUDRA CONCEPT

Part Two
THE MUDRAS

Part Three
PRACTICAL APPLICATIONS

Appendices

SPECIFIC MUDRAS

ACKNOWLEDGMENTS

A person can never really complete a work like this alone. In order to write this book, I relied on the contributions of many other people. Many people helped me in the process of gaining knowledge and perception about mudras in general; and many others helped me with my research on the effects of working with mudras. There are many people I would like to thank for their help in this. Within a few months of beginning this project I "coincidentally" met people who were involved with the mudras either on a scientific and/or practical basis. They had been successfully using mudras for years and generously offered their knowledge for my use. In addition, some of my yoga students tested the mudras and confirmed the findings. From the bottom of my heart, I would like to thank those who helped me.

I sincerely thank *Kim da Silva* for permitting me to use some of his mudras, which have also helped me personally. Moreover, I would like to thank him for his suggestions and additions. Thanks as well to *Elisabeth Steudler* for her tips on herbs. Her knowledge, enthusiasm, and love of plants made my heart feel warm and wide.

I thank *Ito Joyoatmojo,* who drew more than 100 hands. The pictures of the hands on pages 38 and 39 are from G. Hürlimann's *Handlesen* (Wettsbilt). Many thanks also to *Erika Schuler-Konietzny,* for her help with my original manuscript.

DEAR READER

*W*ith this book, I would like to give you and your loved ones (even people who are currently confined to their beds) a practical aid in healing both minor and major complaints. *Mudras: Yoga in Your Hands* is my fourth book, and four is the number for rest, stability, and order. This is why I originally wanted to bring a book about rest and meditation into our loud world. In *Basic Yoga for Everybody,* my third book (and the first translated into English), I presented a few mudras (the special finger or hand positions) for intensifying meditation; and then my German publisher requested that I write a book solely on the topic of mudras. This suggestion suited me quite well, since the very nature of mudras is repose, silence, and peace.

I will even dare to claim that most health disorders, whether on the physical or the mental-emotional level, develop from a lack of inner and outer repose and/or too much stress or worry. Since I personally am all too well acquainted with both outer and inner unrest (and have developed some strategies against it with the help of the mudras) I can consider myself healthy and happy today, in both the physical and the mental-emotional sense. I especially enjoy using the mudras since the effort involved is very minimal. We can practise mudras anywhere, anytime, no matter where we are.

Despite the stress that often rules our lives, we are forced to experience periods of rest from time to time. These rest times are also waiting periods. What happens to your mood when you are sitting in traffic, standing in line at the counter, missing the train, twiddling your thumbs at the computer, laying in bed with the flu or a broken bone, or after preparing a meal and your loved ones aren't home? These can all be times of aggravation, inner conflict, or frustration. (I used to hate waiting for anything.) Or they can become times of regeneration and self-communion.

Today, I find that waiting times forced upon me in a quite incidental way, either by the outside world or from inside myself, have become very precious. They are times of pausing. I can use them to gain fresh insight, create new perspectives, or formulate new principles. In yoga, the inner occurrences and their effects are compared with a lake. In everyday life, thoughts and feelings are always in motion, and these movements can be compared with the waves of a lake. The air (mind) moves the water (soul). If a wind springs up, then waves form. If we look into agitated water, then everything is unclear. Our own face and the surrounding world are distorted and clouds (restless and worried thoughts) cover the sun (symbol of the Divine). If the lake is calm, then we can see down to the bottom. Everything reflected in it is clear and beautiful, and we can once again recognise the sun.

By using the mudras in combination with *breathing exercises, visualisation,* and *affirmation,* I have had wonderful experiences of attaining inner peace and quiet and making the most of the present moment. This is why most of this book consists of these combinations.

I have long been interested in nutrition (so that I can keep asthma and allergies at bay) and herbal remedies. Since I have learned how much our health is dependent upon what we eat, I have included information about food and health in the appendices. However, I wish to present nutrition as a pleasurable addition instead of a dogmatic necessity. Even I am entitled to a little piece of fine chocolate with a tiny cup of espresso! (See Appendix A.)

One or two herbs are mentioned in most of the mudra sections. I have selected them in collaboration with Elisabeth Steudler, an experienced pharmacist who is an authority in the field of herbology. She is full of health and vitality, and looks 15 years younger than she is! That's proof she puts her knowledge to practical use and it works. We have consciously decided against describing special tea recipes since the herbal preparations can also be obtained in the form of tinctures, lozenges, drops, ointments, aroma essences, or in homeopathic form. You will find more on this topic in Appendix B.

I am especially pleased about writing this book because it can help everyone – the average person as well as those who are ill and must stay in bed, or who no longer have the strength to practise the physical exercises of yoga. Many years ago, I was in such a physically weakened state for several months. Because of asthma my energy was so low that I broke into tears at even the thought of trying to lift a cup. I know what it means to be physically, mentally, and emotionally weak. Had I been familiar with this type of book back then, I would have been spared some physical pain and emotional suffering. Since I have been imprinted by such experiences, it has always been a special concern to address both the physical and the mental-emotional realm, as they all work together.

If you would first like to know more about the background and effects of the mudras before working with them, then continue reading here. If you are only interested in the how, where, when, and how much – then continue reading on page 6. You can read this book from cover to cover or you can just look at "Mudras for the Body, Mind, and Soul" to select your own mudras. The individual mudras are described so precisely that you need no additional knowledge to do them. If you are looking for a specific mudra for a certain purpose, such as against headaches, look up this term in the Index. You will find the appropriate mudra for this purpose listed there.

There is one thing you must keep in mind: even though a great deal is written about healing here, this book does not replace a physician. You can approach your health like I do – have your doctor clarify the type of health disorder and make a clear diagnosis. Then try the natural remedies. If these do not have a positive effect, then bring in the heavy artillery, which your doctor will be happy to prescribe for you. Today, most doctors are willing to confer with a mature patient. Two years ago, when I cured pneumonia by using potato compresses and thyme vapour, my doctor ultimately became quite interested in this method. "I congratulate you on the success of your treatment. But how many other people are willing to suffer voluntarily and have the necessary patience?" was his comment.

I hope you enjoy trying out the mudras and the supportive remedies from God's pharmacy presented here. I am certain you will be enthusiastic about the results!

Yours truly,

Gertrud Hirschi

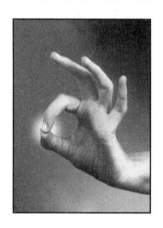

PART ONE

Exploring the
Mudra Concept

WHAT ARE MUDRAS?

*M*udra is a term with many meanings. It is used to signify a gesture, a mystic position of the hands, a seal, or even a symbol. However, there are eye positions, body postures, and breathing techniques that are called mudras. These symbolic finger, eye, and body postures can vividly depict certain states or processes of consciousness. Conversely, specific positions can also lead to the states of consciousness that they symbolise. What does this mean in concrete terms? For example, a person who frequently and fervently does the gesture of fearlessness, which can often be seen in the depiction of Indian deities, will also be freed from fearfulness with time. So mudras engage certain areas of the brain and/or soul and exercise a corresponding influence on them. However, mudras are also effective on the physical level. I discuss this in the section called "Mudras and Other Hand Therapies."

We can effectively engage and influence our body and our mind by bending, crossing, extending, or touching the fingers with other fingers. Isn't this wonderful?

In Hatha Yoga,[1] there are 25 mudras. These also include eye and body positions *(asanas)* and locks *(bandhas)*. In this book, I will only briefly touch on them and mainly describe the hand mudras. Especially in

---

[1] This school of yoga is the most popular in the West. It includes physical exercises, cleansing exercises, and breathing exercises.

Kundalini Yoga,[2] the hand mudras are used during the body postures to intensify their effect. The kundalini expert Lothar-Rüdiger Lütge explains: "In this respect, Kundalini Yoga assumes that every area of the hand forms a reflex zone for an associated part of the body and the brain. In this way, we can consider the hands to be a mirror for our body and our mind."[3]

As I recently meditated on the term *mudra,* I became particularly aware of the symbol of a lock. A lock always conceals a secret. We frequently use gestures in an unconscious way to seal something; for example, when giving special weight to a decision, or reaching an agreement with another person, or even with cosmic consciousness. In precisely the same way, we may also seal something with our inner forces – we reach an understanding with ourselves. I don't believe we will ever completely understand the essence of the mudras. The enigmatic touches on the Divine – so each mudra ultimately creates a special connection to cosmic consciousness (or however you prefer to call the Divine). This symbolism, in particular, is the basis of the best-known hand mudra of yoga, the Chin Mudra.

The thumb is symbolic of cosmic (divine) and the index finger is symbolic of individual (human) consciousness. The ultimate or primary goal of yoga is the oneness of humanity with cosmic consciousness. With this gesture, the human being expresses this desire, this longing. It is

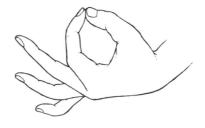

---

[2] The goal of this school of yoga is awakening the spiritual strength that rests in every human being at the lower end of the spinal column and letting it rise up through the spinal column until it unites with the Divine above the top of the head.

[3] Lothar-Rüdiger Lütge, *Kundalini* (Freiburg, 1989), p. 72.

interesting to note that both these fingers belong to the metal element in Chinese Five Element Theory (see Appendix C for more about this topic). Metal is the material that is the best conductor – it conducts energy. According to this teaching, the metal element also creates the connection with the cosmic world, and inspiration and intuition dwell in this element. The index finger represents inspiration (energy from the outside) and the thumb stands for intuition (inner energy). In this gesture, intuition and inspiration form a closed unity. The power of the microcosm and the macrocosm are connected and mutually fructify each other. We see that if we dig into the depths of the ancient teachings long enough – or go far enough into the heights – we will find ourselves at the other end again.

ORIGIN OF MUDRAS

*T*he origin of the mudras is a mystery. Mudras are not only found in Asia, but they are also used throughout the entire world. In their rituals, our European ancestors certainly were familiar with specific gestures, which they used to underline and seal what they thought and wanted to say. During the Christianisation of the Nordic peoples, many gestures were initially prohibited, such as invoking the gods with raised arms. Later, these gestures were partially integrated into the Christian teachings. If we observe the various gestures made by a priest saying the Mass, we can perhaps sense how these ancient peoples expressed themselves. But our everyday life is also characterised by gestures, the origins of which hardly anyone knows today: crossing our fingers for someone, clapping our hands as applause, the handshake, holding hands, or "giving someone the finger" to display our low opinion of them.

In India, mudras are an established component of all religious activities. The various mudras and *hastas* (arm poses) are significant in the depiction of Hindu gods. In addition to body postures and attributes, they also represent the distinguishing characteristics of various deities. The person at prayer sees a special power, capability, and strength of character in these mystical hand poses. The best-known mudras of the major gods Brahma (Creator), Vishnu (Preserver), and Shiva (Destroyer) are numbers 41, 42, 43, 46, 47, and 48.

The mudras are just as familiar in Indian dance, where the hands, eyes, and body movements act and/or dance the entire drama without words. Mudra specialist Ingrid Ramm-Bonwitt describes this beautifully, "The hands are the bearers of important symbols, which are still universally understood in the East today. With his or her hands, the Indian dancer expresses the life of the universe. Through its variety of interpretive possibilities, the rich symbolism of the dance's language of gestures gains a greater significance for the mind than words could express. . . . The spiritual meaning of the mudras found its perfect expression in Indian art. The gestures of the deities depicted in Hindu and Buddhist art . . . symbolise their functions or evoke specific mythological occurrences."[4]

Mudras are also practised in Tantric rituals.[5] They play a large role in Buddhism, where six mudras are very familiar in the pictorial depictions of Gautama Buddha. These are very closely related to his teachings and his life (see mudra numbers 41, 43, 46, 47, 48, and 49).

Hatha Yoga also expresses the many states of mind, such as mourning, joy, anger, and serenity, through gestures and body positions. They realise that the reverse also applies – certain gestures can positively influence the psyche.

How Are Mudras Practised?

Quite simply: Form your hands and place the fingers as they are shown in the various illustrations. When you do this, *the pressure of the fingers should be very light and fine, and your hands should be relaxed*. But perhaps you may notice that this isn't all that simple! The fingers are rebellious, too inflexible, and the hands slip away or tire quickly. The flexibility of the hands has a direct relationship to the flexibility of the entire body. If we are tense at a certain place in the body, this tension will be expressed at a corresponding

---

[4] Ingrid Ramm-Bonwitt: *Mudras – Geheimsprache der Yogis* (Freiburg, 1988), cover.
[5] One of the major doctrines of worshipping God in modern Hinduism. Here mainly Shakti, the wife of the Hindu god Shiva, is worshipped as the "Divine Mother."

area in the hands. Even a person's age can be determined on the basis of the spread fingers – at least this is what the Chinese healing practitioners claim.

My body and my hands have become very flexible through many years of yoga practise. Yet, I can only do the mudra against backaches, which I need the most, with one hand because I have to use the other to hold the fingers in position. At the beginning, you may perhaps also have problems in doing some of the mudras with both hands because you will first have to arrange and hold the fingers of one hand with the other. If this is the case, just do the mudra with the one hand for the time being. If the fingers that should actually be stretched curl on their own again, simply press them onto your thigh or some other place where you can rest them. With time, the tensions will dissolve in the fingers or hand, as well as in the corresponding area of the body.

Do the mudra as well as possible and the effect will appear in any case. In the beginning, it may be difficult to keep the fingers extended. When the fingers get tired, they give in. With time, I am certain that you will gain more strength in your hands, become more flexible, and will be able to use both hands. You will also feel more refreshed and flexible. It is also possible that you will feel somewhat younger.

Even when you have become stronger and more flexible, always treat your fingers in a careful and loving way. It doesn't matter why you are doing the mudra, it should not only be a healing gesture, but also a holy gesture.

Mudras can be done while seated, lying down, standing, and walking. Be sure that your body posture is symmetrical and centred, and that you are as relaxed and loose as possible. If you sit on a chair while doing them, your back should be straight and your feet should have good contact with the floor. If you do them while lying down, resting on your back is naturally the most suitable position. If you stay in this position for a long period of time, put a small pillow beneath the back of your head to take the strain off the neck. To relieve your back, you can put a cushion under the

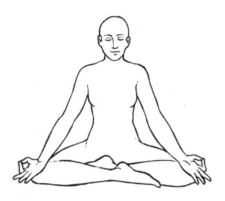

hollow of the knee or thigh. It is important to remain comfortable and relaxed, for any tension will also hinder the inner flow of energy and we want something new to flow with the mudras. If you do them while walking, make sure you move in an even, calm, and rhythmic way. If you stand while doing them, keep your legs shoulder distance apart. The knees should be relaxed, and the tips of the toes must point forward.

If you have a bit more time, you can also do the mudras in a seated meditation position – this will turn them into a longer period of meditation. When you do this, take into consideration the following basic principles of meditation technique:

- Sit with an upright pelvis and a straight spinal column on a stable cushion. Both knees should be flat on the ground or at the same height (if necessary, support the lower knee with a cushion until it is at the same height as the other knee).

- Let the hands relax on the thighs.

- Let the shoulders fall back and down in a relaxed way; your chest should be open and free.

- Pull the chin back a bit, and let the neck be long and relaxed.

- Breathe in an even, slow, flowing, and gentle way.

- Never end the meditation suddenly. Always vigorously stretch your arms and legs.

You can also form a mudra and think of something else at the same time. However, I have found that the effect is accelerated and intensified when you simultaneously assume a meditative position, focus on your hands, and observe your breathing. Observing the normal flow of the breath or influencing and directing the breath is a very important way of supporting the mudra. How to do this is explained for the individual mudras. Corresponding visualisations and affirmations can be used so that this never becomes just a routine matter. These also intensify the effects of the mudras. For some exercises, I am no longer certain what has the greatest effect – the mudra, the breathing technique, the visualised image, or the spoken word. But who cares? It fulfils its purpose, lets you feel good, and makes you happy!

Where and When Can You Practise Mudras?

You can actually practise the mudras at any time and in any place. Modern authors take the view that mudras can even be done while stuck in traffic, watching television, or when you have to wait for someone or something. However, my opinion differs somewhat from this perspective for the following reasons: mudras should be done in a meditative, harmonious mood. Can you guarantee that while stuck in traffic you won't be stressed and fuming with annoyance because you aren't getting to where you want to go, or that you sit in front of the television because you are "relaxing" by watching a hard-core thriller or vehement political debate on taxes?

I invite you to do an interesting test: place your thumb and index finger together and think about something wonderful for a few minutes while you do this (an experience in nature, winning at sports, sex, etc.) – it doesn't matter what it is, as long as it lets you float on pink clouds. Now try to feel the energy that flows from the index finger to the thumb. Finished! Now do the same thing again, but this time imagine something terribly sad. Once again, feel the energy of the fingers. Do you notice a difference? You will certainly have discovered how dull the flow of energy felt the second time.

This little experiment shows me how important it is to practise mudras while in a good mood and in a positive atmosphere. Feelings and thoughts influence the energy fields and the flow of energy in a negative or positive manner, even if we don't notice it. This is no joking matter. As I will explain later, we want to engage these energy fields in a positive sense. This is why the basic tone of our momentary mood and situation is so important. However, there are also mudras and breathing techniques for serenity, patience, and composure. These can be used to initially get into the right mood. For example, when stuck in traffic, standing in line, or sitting on a train, we can first calm down and then begin practising the actual mudra.

When holding a mudra while watching television or listening to the radio, one further factor should be taken into consideration – the time we spend on a mudra should always be a time of self-communion as well. The only exceptions are special programmes or music with a much more calming than stimulating effect on the nerves. If we have planned our days so poorly that we don't have three peaceful minutes, if we let ourselves constantly be exposed to the radio or television from our first waking moments until we fall asleep at night, then mudras actually have no place in our lives.

Mudras can truly be practised almost anywhere and at any time, but only when we can also withdraw within ourselves almost anywhere and at any time. This really isn't all that difficult and can be learned, like everything else. It concerns our health – we need a few silent minutes now and then every day. These silent moments can be the most precious to us; and like the salt in the dough that gives the bread its good taste, silence adds the right spice to our lives.

A good time to practise mudras is a few minutes before getting up and a few minutes before falling asleep, before or after meals, when you walk somewhere (we all need to walk a certain distance every day), while on public transportation, or during breaks at work.

However, don't just try out a number of mudras in a row at random. Specifically select just one or two. Practise these according to a time plan. Decide when, how long, and how often you want to do them every day. Or plan to fill both the usual and unpredictable times with them when you have to wait. Practise only these mudras over the next few days. The effects may occur immediately, especially if you have acute complaints or mood swings. But it may also be that the effects you hope for only occur after several days. For chronic complaints, it usually takes several weeks or even months before an improvement takes place. Only patience can help here. Moreover, it is always worth it since many new perceptions can be gained and wonderful moments experienced, in addition to the desired healing. You should also know that when something changes within, there is a corresponding change in your surrounding world.

Every healing within also brings healing into your world. An illness in the body is always connected with thoughts and feelings that make people sick. A certain amount of time is required before healing takes place on every level. So allow yourself the time – practise ardently and remain completely serene and confident while doing so. Then the chances of healing will be the greatest.

How Long is a Mudra Held?

The great masters do not agree on the length of time to practise a mudra position. The Indian mudra researcher Keshav Dev recommends holding one mudra per day for 45 minutes; chronic complaints can be eliminated in this way.[6] If it isn't possible to do this, these 45 minutes can be divided into three time periods of 15 minutes each. The kinesiologist Kim da Silva,

---

[6] I have taken this and all of the following information from Keshav Dev on the effect of the mudras from the article "Yoga mit dem kleinen Finger" by Ram Panjaabi in the German magazine *esotera* 9/88.

who has tested the effect of mudras over longer periods of time, recommends an individually, precisely determined time for holding each mudra. If you use a mudra as support for some type of therapy or to heal a *chronic* complaint, then I think it is beneficial to use it routinely, like a medication: every day at the same time and for the same length of time.

Mudras that are used for *acute* complaints – such as respiratory and circulation problems, flatulence, exhaustion, or inner restlessness – should be discontinued when the appropriate effect is achieved. Other mudras can be practised for 3 to 30 minutes, two to four times a day. Using a stopwatch is the ideal way to time them. The time specifications that I have assigned to the individual mudras are meant to be an orientation aid, but not a dogma. You will also notice that your hands, especially the fingers, will become increasingly sensitive and respond to the mudras much more quickly after they have been given some training. If you need 5 minutes at the start to feel the effect of a mudra, in time you will only need 10 breaths. This is a wonderful experience! However, if you are confined to your bed, then you have enough time and should permit yourself to make good use of it. Also let the visualisations and affirmations continue to have their lasting effect afterward. You can use this time for your own benefit, for the healing of the body, mind, and soul.

The effect of a mudra may be perceived immediately or only after a certain amount of time. You start to feel warm, the sense of unwellness and pain fade away, your mood improves, and your mind is refreshed. But exactly the opposite may occur at the start. You become tired, or start to feel cold and shiver. This is also a positive sign of the effect.

BREATHING, VISUALISATION, AND AFFIRMATIONS TO ENHANCE THE MUDRAS

*T*he effect of a mudra can be immensely intensified with the breath. This is why it is very important to know what breathing does. When you understand the following principles, then you can influence the effect of a mudra according to your own needs.

- Pay attention to a symmetrical posture and hold your arms about one inch away from your body. Even this position alone brings a sense of inner equilibrium and harmony as it regulates the activity of the nervous system and hormonal glands.

- In addition to carbon dioxide, we also discharge expended energy on the subtle level when we exhale deeply. This is why you should always exhale vigorously several times at the beginning of a mudra. Make room for what you want to achieve.

- **Always lengthen the little pause after inhaling and after exhaling by several seconds.** This is the most important aspect of the breathing process. The inner powers are developed during the pauses – on every level.

- When you practise a mudra *to calm yourself,* then *slow your breathing.*

- When you practise a mudra to *refresh* yourself, then *intensify your breathing*.

- The optimal quality of breathing is achieved when the breath is slow, deep, rhythmic, flowing, and fine.

At the beginning of a mudra meditation, exhale vigorously several times and then let the breath become deeper and slower. You now have three possibilities:

First: Focus on your hands and fingers, perceive the gentle pressure where they touch each other;

Second: While inhaling, you can press the fingertips together a bit more and let go of the pressure when exhaling;

Third: You can do it the other way around and apply a bit more pressure while exhaling and let go of the pressure when inhaling.

Every variation has its special effect. The first variation centres, creates inner equilibrium, and builds up strength in general. The second variation strengthens the will and refreshes. The third variation calms and relaxes. Try out these variations and feel the difference yourself! It is possible that you won't immediately feel the effect, but it is still there.

The outer circumstances of our lives usually shape themselves according to our imagination and the contents of our minds. So we have the possibility of shaping our inner images in such a way that we enjoy life, experience success in our work, and have relationships on a loving and understanding basis. It is very important to create an unshakable faith and be filled with both fervour and serenity to accompany our self-made images. We need to create little experiences of success for ourselves, since what functions in a small way will also succeed on a larger scale. We can slowly build and develop this confidence. Just imagine what would happen if a great many people would simultaneously imagine a beautiful world with rich flora, content animals, happy human beings, and firmly believe that this is possible. Join in – then there will already be two of us!

If we can clearly express what we do not want and definitively formulate our wishes and needs, this can already be the beginning of a new order in life. For many years now, I have worked with affirmations – sometimes more, sometimes less. Time and time again, their astounding effects have astonished me. For example, my kitten disappeared one day. I repeated the same sentence over and over the entire day: "With divine strength and power, I find my kitten again." Toward evening, I simply knew where my kitten was. The woman was completely perplexed when I claimed that my cat was in her garage, but it was true. It is so simple, and some people even find it a bit naive. But things that are particularly simple and naive usually have the greatest effective power.

The same principle applies to affirmations as it does to visualisations. Say them full of faith, fervour, and serenity. You can say them one to three times, during or after the meditation. You can also pause for a moment during the day and speak your affirmation in a quiet or a loud voice. Make use of this wonderful possibility and talk yourself into what you really want – what is good for you.

If you want to get rid of something stubborn, a negation can also be helpful. Speak it at the beginning, while you are vigorously exhaling. For example, "This hatred (or resentment, feeling of guilt, pain, fear, desire to smoke, etc.) will immediately disappear and dissolve itself."

MUDRAS AND MUSIC

Some clinics and rehabilitation centres use music as a component of routine therapy. We all know the healing effect of music, as a number of books have been published on the subject. But music is also good for healthy people who are occasionally plagued by weakness or physical imbalances. Since the music used for therapy plays anywhere from three to twelve minutes, and this amount of time corresponds to how long one holds a mudra, it is obvious that mudras and music can have a wonderful influence on each other. Tension – either physical or mental-emotional – can be relieved by listening to the right kind of music. The right kind of music has a calming and relaxing effect, possibly even taking a person into a state of deep relaxation. Stress and tension can also lead to an acute or a chronic state of exhaustion that can be positively influenced by music.

If you pay attention to the following points, you can get a lot from using music with your mudras:

- Consider your own taste in music;

- Determine how long the playing time should be;

- Listen to the same piece at the same time for at least three days in row;

- Listen consciously, and immediately let go of any thoughts that may arise.

Which music pieces are best suited for this purpose? Helen Bonny, who developed GIM (Guided Imagery Music), writes: "Tranquilising and relaxing music is oriented to the human heart, on a calm and relaxed pulse. Overall, tranquilising music is distinctly calm and more harmonious, with lightly flowing melodies. A person doesn't have to immediately fall asleep to it, but this music promotes specific feelings, such as an inner calm, relaxation, and contentment."[7]

According to the opinion of the GIM trainer, classical music is particularly suited for healing and relaxing, and solo concerts have a stronger effect than symphonies. There is a special power in slow movements – andante, adagio, and largo. For a relaxation effect, the most suitable instrument is the oboe, followed by the piano, the cello, the violin, the clarinet, and the organ. Vocals are less suited for promoting relaxation. The following keys are the most effective: C major, D major, B major, and F major. In summary, it can be said that many low and few high frequencies lead to relaxation. High frequency, "airy" music tends to be more suited for a light, elevating mood. With these guidelines, you can now put together your own appropriate and individual music pharmacy.

It is worthwhile to find out which music especially appeals to you so you can become more conscious of your own individuality in this respect. For example, some relaxation music has precisely the opposite effect on me – it gets on my nerves, and even makes me feel aggressive.

Incidentally, if you have trouble taking the time to do chores around the house, try playing some snappy marches or hot rock music, or even techno, to bring fresh momentum into this bothersome situation!

---

[7] Lutz Berger: "Die Magie der heilenden Klänge" in *esotera* 6/97, p. 27.

MUDRAS AND COLOUR

Colours influence our minds and our lives on every level. In colour therapy, various shades of colour are specifically applied to regenerate the organs and glands, as well as to activate the processes of elimination, respiration, and circulation. Colours also influence our moods and every type of mental activity.

- **Red** stimulates the circulation, makes us alert, warms and relaxes, but can also bring out aggression;

- **Orange** improves the mood, promotes lightness, stimulates sexuality, but can also stimulate superficiality;

- **Yellow** stimulates digestion, makes us mentally alert, and lets life appear in a bright light, but it can also be obtrusive;

- **Green** is generally calming; it regenerates on every level, and gives us the desire to start something new;

- **Blue** is also calming, but this calmness goes deeper and provides a sense of security; it conveys protection, and symbolises the silent yearning for the incomprehensible;

- **Violet** is the colour of transformation, change, and spirituality;

- **Brown** is the colour of stability and connection to the earth, but too much can lead to stagnation;

- **White** bears the entire spectrum of the other colours within itself, containing birth as well as death;

- **Black** is the colour of protection, of gathering strength, of retreat, and of the emptiness that already bears abundance within itself. Many teenagers like to wear black because they stand at the gateway of a new period of their lives. However, too much black weakens the organism, puts us in a sad mood, and promotes pessimism.

There are basically no "bad" colours, but it is important to use the right proportions. Every colour can also be seen in our aura or energy body. When a colour gains dominance or is not in its right place, it will initially have an effect on the general feeling of well-being. With time, a health disorder may develop as a result. However, the course of an illness can also be reversed with the help of colours.

It would go beyond the scope of this book to discuss the entire spectrum of colours used in healing. The following suggestions can help you have some good and beautiful experiences using colour meditations. If you prefer a certain colour, it may well be that you need the corresponding qualities. However, if you give too much preference to one colour, this can develop into an addiction and the colour may harm you.

While holding a mudra, you can either visualise a colour or concentrate on the colour of an object. The first approach is better because the colour will then come to life, which means you can imagine the colour as dark or light, dull or bright, connected to forms, or flowing, etc. For example, you feel the need to go into the forest because you can best regenerate yourself there but don't have the time to do so. You can imagine a very green forest, and in your thoughts, you can totally luxuriate in the green of the leaves. This will refresh you inwardly. Such visualisations have long been used successfully, and pictures of lush landscapes are specifically installed in many hospitals to support the healing process. Try it out!

USING MUDRAS TO HEAL
PHYSICAL COMPLAINTS

*M*udras used against a great variety of health disorders are primarily found in Chinese medicine. These usually have their origin in the Five Element Theory (see Appendix C), the principles of which are still unknown in the West. However, the Indian yoga master and healer Keshav Dev, who intensively researched the effect of the mudras many years ago, can also confirm the healing power of the mudras. He says: "Your destiny lies in your hands, and this should be taken quite literally. Not only because the hand lines show the past and future of a person, but above all because each finger has its very own functions and power within the organism. If you know how to use this power, you can maintain your physical health and mental peace. When I tell patients about the mudras, their first reaction is skepticism. They ask me, 'How can my illness be improved if I do nothing more than just press together a few of my fingers?' But as soon as they begin to trust and have carried out the exercises, they feel the effect and their skepticism changes into astonishment. Then I explain to them that these techniques, which look so simple, are extremely valuable gifts that were given to us from the most enlightened yoga masters of ancient times."[8]

---

[8] Keshav Dev, "Yoga mit dem Kleinen Finger," by Ram Panjaabi in *esotera* 9/98.

Everyone who has been involved with the healing effect of the mudras emphasises that a sensible lifestyle and diet must absolutely be taken into consideration. An unhealthy lifestyle usually consists of inferior diet, lack of exercise, and too little fresh air, rest, and relaxation – coupled with too much stress, worry, negative thoughts, and negative feelings. Practising the mudras, together with a healthy diet, routine rest periods, adequate exercise (yoga, jogging, hiking, biking, etc.) will naturally lead to an optimal lifestyle. And this is the basis for health. (Also see Appendix A.)

When mudras are used to support the healing of chronic health disorders, they should be routinely employed as a course of treatment over a period of several weeks or months. A chronic disease has already had its beginnings within a person many years before it actually becomes evident. Consequently, a certain amount of time is required in order to dissolve the waste materials that have deposited themselves in the arteries, organs, individual cells, and energy fields.

Some mudras can also be used as **help in an emergency** (for example: lumbago, dizziness, nausea, or heart attack). Practise these when they are necessary and only as long as they are necessary. Sudden complaints are not a coincidence, but are the explosion of an imbalanced state that has already flared up within us for a longer period of time. This is why a mudra shouldn't just be used like a fast-acting medication to subdue symptoms. Get to the bottom of the matter. Meditate – ask inside yourself what this physical attack means for you. Ask persistently and honestly, for then you will also receive an honest answer. Perhaps it won't be comfortable, but it will have a healing effect in the long run.

MUDRAS AND HEALING EMO-
TIONAL PROBLEMS

*O*ne important reason why I started with yoga was an experience I
had as a young person taking asthma medication. As a result of taking medication, I could no longer grasp correlations, and my memory was impaired; I was apathetic and immensely indifferent. I thought I
might be "sick in the head" and might stay that way. Since then, I have been
interested in brain research and everything that keeps people mentally fit.
Mudras do true wonders in this field. For a number of years now, hand exercises have been successfully used on children in special education classes.

Run your thumb along your fingertips in a gentle and conscious way.
This feels wonderful! It's refreshing for your brain. The brain should be
trained like a muscle every day. It has been proved that even after a few
days of rest in bed (after an operation, for example), the activity of the brain
is reduced. It has also been demonstrated that the brain can regenerate very
quickly through the appropriate training. Practising mudras can be called
pure brain training. There is a positive influence on the brain waves, particularly when the fingertips touch each other. When we visualise inner
images at the same time, this requires a great deal of ability from the brain
and promotes the power of the imagination. This power is one of the preconditions for mental alertness and clear thinking.

The accompanying affirmations promote a clear manner of expression, which is also a mental power. When a mudra is done with full

concentration, and a state of serenity is maintained, cerebral activity is calmed and regenerated. In addition, many mudras synchronise the right and left hemisphere of the brain. This promotes memory, the general ability to recollect, and, miraculously, creativity as well.

I will risk claiming that a trained brain remains fit up into a ripe old age. The great yogis have also demonstrated this to us with their mental alertness as seniors. I can also observe – and my surrounding world has confirmed this – that my own ability to recollect, my memory, clear thinking, and concentration have never been so pronounced as today. Colleagues who are as old as I am complain about the opposite. And I am no more talented than they are! The only difference is that I constantly train my brain.

Always see the good in your fellow human beings, put the negative aspects of the past behind you, live completely in the present, and make the best you possibly can of it. Expect the best from the future and remain in constant contact with cosmic consciousness – then nothing will stand in the way of a meaningful and happy life.

I can hardly describe the blessings that this kind of constructive thinking has brought me. Incidentally, this attitude in life is also the best for my health.

Mudras have a wondrous effect on the *emotional area* of our lives, which includes the soul, our feelings, and our moods. It is no coincidence that people make fists when they are vehemently agitated, or that hands become limp and their movements flighty during depressions. If we want to change oppressive moods, we can do so by changing our breathing rhythm accordingly. The way we breathe can stimulate us, calm us, inflame us, or cool us down.

Mood fluctuations, which many people suffer from today, can often be largely eliminated within a few days by using mudras. However, I recommend that you practise the respective mudra and meditation three times a day for at least 10 minutes (or twice for 20 minutes) while lying down or sitting.

Moods and physical complaints are similar. In order to cure them, we must look for and remedy the cause, which almost always lies *within*. We should never blame our surrounding world for our moods. Parents, children, partners, colleagues at work – they are only reflections of our inner life. Even if we initially can't change our environment, we can work on our inner attitude toward the surrounding world, changing it in small steps.

Perhaps your response to this is, "But I worry." Does it help you in any way to worry? Does worry improve your circumstances? I know how difficult it is to let go of worry. Conversations to clear up the situation and/or a prayer have always helped me the most in dealing with them. The divine powers have always helped me up to now – without exception. Each of you will be helped, if you only permit it. When you let go of a worry, you no longer have to think about it.

Chronic bad moods of any type (aggression, depression, dissatisfaction, fear, etc.) can also be caused by weakened or even sick organs, digestive problems, blood pressure, pain, or other physical reasons. As you practise the mudras used for physical healing, these moods may be remedied to a large extent. Meditation, visualisation, and affirmation all have a positive effect on the mental-emotional area. If you are attentive to this, you can watch how the positive changes of your mood tread softly as they slip into your life. You will be more content, serene, courageous, and cheerful. Just wait – this is what will happen!

MUDRAS AND OTHER HAND THERAPIES

*W*e will never completely comprehend the magnificent correlations of our world. There is an order – on both a large and small scale – a reason for this universe of ours. Relationships and correspondences fill me with awe.

For example, can you imagine what it means when scientists claim that the code of the entire body, including character traits, is inherent to the nucleus of each individual cell? Eastern sages and doctors say that the body, mind, and soul are inherent to every fingertip, every finger joint in each individual finger, and naturally also in the entire hand itself. So it is quite likely that we actually have great influence on every area of the body through the fingers and/or hands.

The effect of mudras will be expressed on many different levels. The physical level is associated with material energy, but the many subtle levels are far from being completely researched. Each human being is an individual energy field or sphere. (To imagine this, think of various coloured swaths of fog that mix together, permeate each other, yet still remain unified within their own colour.) There are different opinions as to how many levels of energy resonate within: some schools speak of five, others of seven, and others of twelve, but there are probably even more.

These energy fields are subject to various vibrations, some of which move more quickly than the others. The physical senses are oriented toward one very specific vibration, and this is why we can only perceive this vibration in particular. However, the ancient yogis could perceive other vibrations, such as those of the *chakras* (energy transformers) and the *nadis,* subtle streams of energy. (If you are not yet familiar with chakra theory, see Appendix D.) In Ayurveda, the healing art that originated in India, the fingers have long had the individual organs and elements associated with them. The Chinese researched the system of meridians, the subtle energy streams, creating various treatment approaches as a result. The Gypsies are said to have developed palmistry, and the hands and individual fingers are also associated with the planetary powers in astrology.

Let's look at the very concrete effect that the hands and fingers have on other areas of the body. There is a direct relationship between the hands and the neck since the nerve paths run through the vertebral foramina in the arms, hands, and fingers. The flexibility of the hands always effects the flexibility of the neck. Therefore, hand exercises relieve tensions in the neck.

Moreover, spreading the ten fingers creates a reflex that causes the thoracic (chest) vertebrae to spread out. This increases the tidal volume of the lungs.

The hands and/or fingers also have an additional direct relationship to the heart and lungs. With increasing age, many people can no longer properly stretch their fingers. This shows tension in the heart area, which often indicates the prelude to heart disease or a tendency toward osteoporosis. This slightly crooked hand position also impedes inhalation. The result is that the optimum amount of air is not drawn into the lungs, especially into the lung borders, which promotes contamination in those areas.

A Little Exercise as a Break

While inhaling, hold your hands in front of your chest with fingers spread. Hold your breath and stretch out your arms horizontally at your side. Now exhale and vigorously make a fist with each hand. Then breathe normally, open the fists, and lower your arms. Repeat three times.

This little exercise expands the bronchial tubes, opens the lungs, strengthens the heart, and refreshes the mind. Asthmatic patients often cough during this exercise because it loosens the mucus in the bronchial tubes, and heart patients feel an intensified awareness of the heart.

Ilse Middendorf, a leading expert in the field of respiratory therapy, has proved that a direct relationship can be established between the individual fingers and the corresponding areas of the lungs. The index fingers and thumbs influence breathing in the upper area of the lungs, the middle finger in the middle area, and the little finger in the lower lung region. You can confirm this statement yourself by placing the tips of the ring finger and little finger on top of each other. Where do you feel the respiratory impulse in particular? Sometimes this test works the first time you try it – otherwise, it usually works after the first few attempts.

Furthermore, the ends of the nerve paths of the hands, as well as the feet, occupy a particularly large area in the brain. This area is much larger than that of the arms and legs. Cerebral activity is activated and trained by touching and feeling, especially with the fingertips. For example, finger games are employed to remedy children's learning difficulties. These games stimulate the corresponding connections in the brain and activate the brain waves. When mudras are practised consciously, which means that we focus on our fingers and whatever they are resting on, they activate large areas of the brain.

Isn't it wonderful that a mudra can have so many positive effects?

Not only can we use mudras to influence all of our body regions and functions, but every act of touching and every movement of the hands has its special effect. Doing handicrafts, playing an instrument, washing the hands, or massaging – all of these acts have long-lasting effects.

- Particularly when you wash your hands, you can squeeze them vigorously and massage them at the same time: Press the four fingers of one hand together with the other hand and turn the fingers you are holding to both sides. Then make fists, open the hands again, and spread the fingers. Or vigorously rub both palms together.

- Or cross your fingers with each other, turn the palms outward, and stretch your arms. This will refresh you, improve your breathing, and strengthen your heart.

- If you sit at a desk for a longer period of time and your neck becomes tense or painful, use the thumb and index finger (with the thumb touching the inside of the hand) to grasp each one of the eight finger-webs at the root of the fingers. Massage the point beneath it and pull the web to the front at least 6 times. When you do this, be sure to be in an upright and relaxed posture.

- If you place the index finger, middle finger, and ring finger of one hand on the longitudinal grooves of the back of the other hand and gently massage back and forth, this will have a regulating effect on the blood pressure.

- A pleasant game to improve your mood, refresh you in a holistic way, and stimulate every bodily function is hand tapping (it is hard to stay serious when you do this, and children can't seem to get enough of it). Clap or tap your hands at least eight times in rhythm. At first, clap in the usual way. Then let the hands hang down and clap the backs of the hands together, then the backs of the fingers, the fingertips, the outer side of the hand, the inner side of the hand, the wrists, the knuckles, etc. The only limit is your imagination. Now you will notice that depending on what you are tapping or how you are clapping, a different tone is created. Use your hands to play your own drum concert. Drumming has been used since time immemorial to initiate healing processes. Today, people are using it for this same purpose again.

With a bit of imagination, you can put together your own programme of hand exercises. You can't do anything wrong here if you carry out every movement slowly and consciously.

The following illustrations will show you various traditions that work with hand energy. This isn't meant to confuse you, but to show you how tremendously diverse this system is. If you take an exact look at it, you will even come across logical inconsistencies. These occur because the individual systems engage various levels, connected like threads that get lost in mysterious unfathomableness – and probably interconnect there.

Ayurveda

People trained in this Indian art of healing consider every illness to be an imbalance within the human body. Healing can take place when the natural balance has been restored. They recognise that the conscious mind creates the disease and that consciousness is an energy that manifests itself in the five basic principles, or elements. If there is too much or too little of any one element, an imbalance occurs (disease). This is restored through corresponding measures. The Chinese also have their Five Element Theory (see Appendix C). However, it takes expert knowledge to reconcile these two systems with each other. Working out the mutual characteristics and the differences would go beyond the scope of this book.

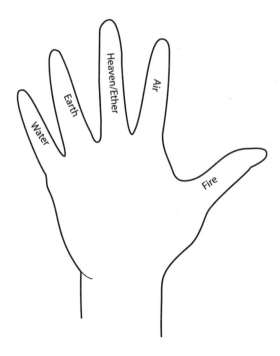

Chakras

The classification of the chakras with the fingers is not the same in all schools of yoga. The most prevalent classification is shown on the hand illustrated here. But there are also yoga masters who classify the *little finger* with the root chakra, the *ring finger* with the sacral chakra, the *middle finger* with the solar plexus chakra, the *index finger* with the heart chakra, and the *thumb* with the throat chakra. It should be noted that only the five chakras found along the spinal column are assigned to the individual fingers. You will find more information about the chakras in Appendix B.

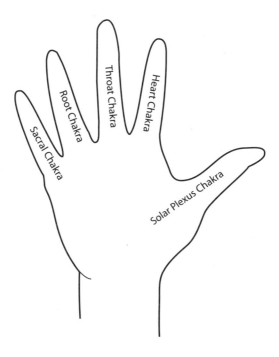

Acupressure

Next to acupuncture, acupressure is the best-known Chinese healing method in the Western countries. Instead of using needles, the meridians are stimulated with the fingers. In the following two illustrations you can see the corresponding points. The nonexpert can simply press them lightly with the thumb for several minutes to achieve a positive effect.

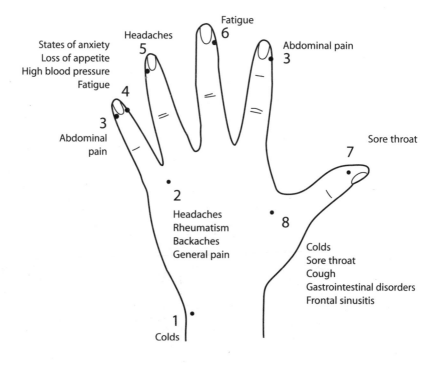

Back of the hand

If you have high blood pressure, massage the middle finger from the root to the tip. To counteract low blood pressure, massage the middle finger from the tip to the root. Do the same with the index finger if you have diarrhea or constipation.

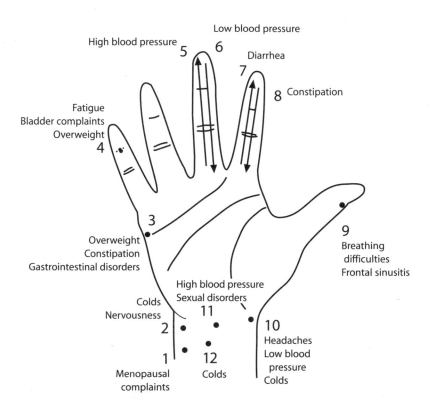

Palm of the hand

Reflex Zones

The hand reflex zones correspond to the foot reflex zones, the massage treatment of which is generally known today. Both of the following illustrations show the reflex points or surfaces that are connected with the muscles and organs. Since some of the organs are only found on one side of the body (such as the heart and liver), this is reflected in the hands.

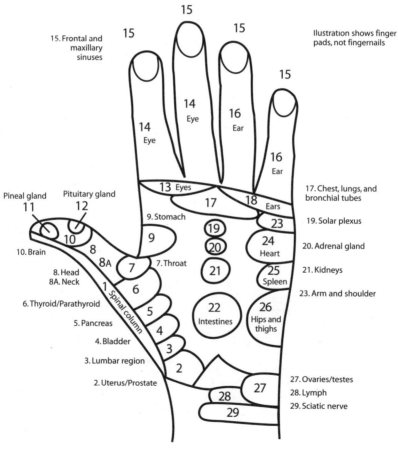

Palm of the hand

Since hands come in different sizes, you may not find the exact pressure point immediately. But with some practise, even the nonexpert can find the right spot.

When you have found the desired point, massage it with your thumb, using light pressure and slow, circular movements. One to 3 minutes are enough.

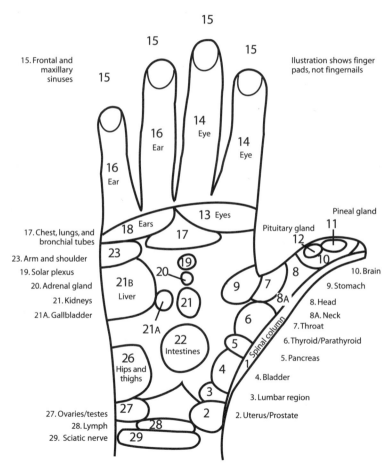

15. Frontal and maxillary sinuses

Ilustration shows finger pads, not fingernails

16. Ear

14. Eye

13. Eyes

Pineal gland

Pituitary gland

17. Chest, lungs, and bronchial tubes
23. Arm and shoulder
19. Solar plexus
20. Adrenal gland
21. Kidneys
21A. Gallbladder

21B. Liver

22. Intestines

Spinal column

10. Brain
9. Stomach
8. Head
8A. Neck
7. Throat
6. Thyroid/Parathyroid
5. Pancreas
4. Bladder
3. Lumbar region
2. Uterus/Prostate

26. Hips and thighs

27. Ovaries/testes
28. Lymph
29. Sciatic nerve

Palm of the hand

Meridians and Deep Meridians

Meridians are the energy paths that run through the body and control its individual functions (circulation, respiration, digestion, and individual organs). The beginning and ending points of the meridians are taken into particular consideration by the mudras. In acupuncture, only the superficial meridians are considered and the system of deep meridians is often even rejected as being speculative. Since the effect of many mudras only

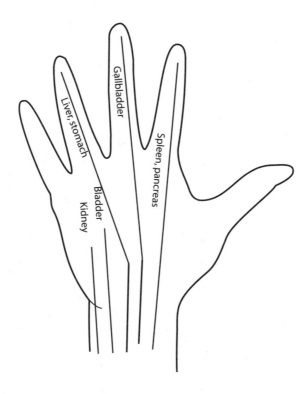

became clear to me once I learned about the deep meridians, I am also presenting this system here.

Try encircling your fingers around your little finger more often. This is good for your heart! If you tend to be chilled easily, or susceptible to illness, then encircle or massage your ring finger.

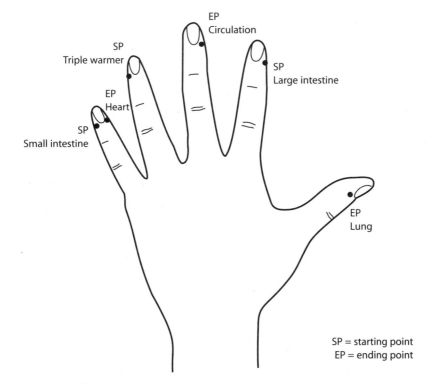

EP
Circulation

SP
Triple warmer

EP
Heart

SP
Small intestine

SP
Large intestine

EP
Lung

SP = starting point
EP = ending point

Planetary Classification and Palmistry

Astrology and palmistry have always belonged together. If the practise of the mudras stimulates your interest in palmistry, you can find a large selection of literature on the topic. The mudras can actually strengthen the hands and the individual fingers, even changing character traits in the process. In the *little finger,* we find creativity, a sense of beauty, and inner clarity; in the *ring finger,* there is sense of family, the ability to love, and a feeling of security; initiative, sobriety, and the love of order are found in the

Astrology

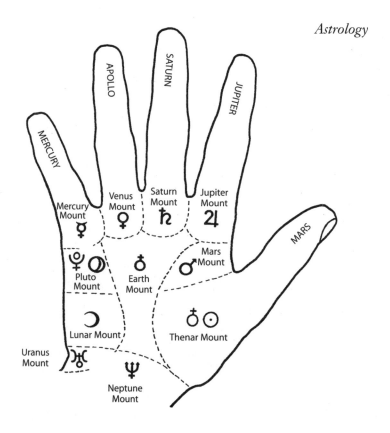

middle finger; intellectual faculty, individuality, and striving for power are in the *index finger;* the will, instinctiveness, and vitality in general are found in the *thumb*. Further classifications from astrology and palmistry can be found in the illustrations on page 38 and the one below.[9]

As you can see, you have "a great deal in your hands" with the mudras. You can take hold of your life with your own two hands and decide what is important to you.

Palmistry

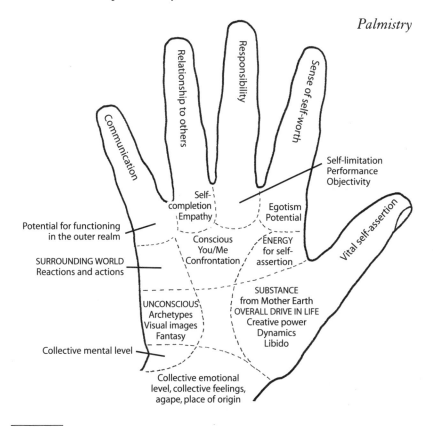

[9] From G. Hürlimann's *Handlesen* (St. Gallen: Wettswil, 1996), pp. 251, 268.

MY PERSONAL EXPERIENCES

*F*or many years, I have successfully used mudras to help me concentrate better or to intensify my meditation. Don't ask me why, but I always felt my little finger games to be something quite intimate, and consequently omitted them from the curriculum of my courses. It probably wasn't the right time for them yet.

At a workshop for brain training several years ago, I became acquainted with Mudra Number 27 and immediately put it to use for a great many different occasions. If I lose the thread while speaking or writing, or if I want to remember something, I simply place the fingertips of both hands together. Then the sentence or word usually comes to mind. Mudra Number 42, the hands placed together in front of the chest, calms my thoughts and supports concentration.

I was also able to counter physical complaints with mudras. One of the most wonderful experiences occurred when I had to lie down after returning from a very long hike. I was very tired and had met a number of people on horseback (I react allergically to the smell of horses), as well as blossoming trees, during the last three miles. This was enough to cause an asthma attack. I did Mudra Number 4, and after four minutes, my breathing was back to normal. I also frequently use Mudra Number 5 when I notice that my chest has become constricted. Perhaps I should do a serious course of treatment at some point using this mudra. During the last flu attack, I often felt wretched. Mudra Number 3, the first version, helped me. Before I go on a long hike, I like to move my bowels, which is done easily if I have already done Mudra Number 23, followed immediately by Mudra 24, while still resting in bed. Fellow hikers also report success with these mudras.

In case of seasickness, or when generally suffering from flatulence after too much fat at a meal, I use Mudra Number 3, the first version, with much success. I find Mudra Number 2 to be great because it practically throws me out of the bed in the morning. It is wonderfully refreshing and counteracts sensations of dizziness.

After a long session of garden work that was followed by an annoying backache, I recently had an interesting experience. I laid down on my back, pulled my knees up to my chest, and did Mudra 17 to balance out the energy in my back. After a few breaths, I felt wonderful and a pleasant warmth flowed through the lumbar vertebral area into my back. I could directly feel how the backache slowly dissolved. Our health and well-being are greatly dependent upon an optimal flow of energy, and tension blocks this energy flow.

Since I am basically a healthy person, it naturally hasn't been possible for me to try out the effects of all of the mudras. However, many of my yoga students and acquaintances have told me about improvement or even the miraculous healing of some conditions. One woman thought that mudras saved her husband's life one night when he woke up with vehement heart pain. She attempted to contact a physician and placed his hands into the form of Mudra 16 while waiting. The heart pain subsided, he fell asleep exhausted, and it wasn't necessary for the physician on emergency call to come immediately. In the morning, she took her husband to the doctor. The diagnosis was that the man had suffered a severe heart attack during the night.[10]

---

[10] Publisher's Note: If you feel heart pain, please get to the emergency room in your hospital. Call an ambulance; make sure you have emergency phone numbers available for quick reference in case you need them. Doing the mudras while waiting for an ambulance is fine. The woman in this story is very lucky that her husband lived through this experience! The mudra exercises do not replace the care of a competent physician.

Another woman thought that her vision had greatly improved with Mudra Number 6. An acquaintance reported considerable success with Mudra 29, which she used for circulatory complaints, and another woman improved her chronic frontal sinusitis with Mudra Number 18.

Many more reports of success could be listed here, but I believe these examples will give you a sense of the wonderful effectiveness of the mudras.

MUDRAS AND MEDITATION

*J*ust like Christian prayer expresses itself through words and corresponding gestures, the Eastern religions also use gestures, mudras, to support the prayer. The meaning and purpose of meditation are also supported by the mudras. In this respect, the Hindus have developed a very differentiated and complete system. In fact, it is so complicated and elaborate that many believers can no longer cope with it and require the help of a priest.

Meditation, as I understand and practise it, has become an indispensable aid in my life. I use it at any time, and everywhere, for everything. As a result, I bring clarity, light, and lightness into my life. I recharge my inner batteries and solve my problems, make decisions, get advice and comfort, refine my character traits, mobilise my immune forces, develop visions for the future – and seek my connection with the Divine. We can use meditation for everything, which includes dissolving anything that bothers, burdens, or annoys us, as well as achieving inner and outer wealth – and naturally also for achieving our spiritual goals. Let's make full use of these possibilities!

Mudras for Recharging Energy Reserves

Whenever you feel listless, tired, or even a bit depressed, many of the mudras can do true wonders. On the one hand, this is true because you permit yourself the well-deserved rest you need and, on the other hand, energy is built up in a very concrete way (which can even be measured).

The following mudras have an especially stimulating and restorative effect: 2, 3, 4, 6, 13, 21, 22, 27, 28, 29, 31, 35, 36, and 39.

Mudras for Coming to Terms with the Past

If we want contentment and peace in our everyday lives, there is no way to avoid clearing out what has burdened us in the past. This doesn't mean looking at the past over and over – but the opposite. We can free ourselves from old resentments, anger, prejudices, feelings of guilt – from everything that weighs on us. The best means to achieve this is forgiveness – forgiving the other person and forgiving yourself. But perhaps we cannot do this alone. Then we can ask our inner wisdom, our higher self, or the Divine within us, for help. Forgiveness, according to Jesus and founders of other great religions, is the most difficult thing, but the best path to finding inner peace. Even if we can just manage to forgive a little, and in time to forgive a little more, then the gateway to a new, light-filled future will open for us. We have only truly forgiven our fellow human beings and ourselves when we can imagine them to be happy and wish them all good things and much love from the depths of our hearts. We must often go through a great deal of pain to achieve this goal.

Mudras 12, 32, 42, and 47 can help accelerate this process of working through and dissolving old feelings.

Mudras for Improving Relationships

Our fellow human beings are our mirror! What we particularly like in others is what we also love within ourselves. What we don't like about others, we also reject within ourselves. We will encounter the same people over and over until we have learned this lesson. When we are ready, the people in our lives will change accordingly, or will disappear from our environment, and others will take their place. This may sound hard, but it is unfortunately true. Isn't it true that other people frequently live out what we don't permit ourselves to do? Some people annoy us with their behaviour. Perhaps they are premature in their judgments, verbally attack others, are hurtful in their thoughtlessness, don't really listen, make us nervous with their restlessness, think they know it all better, are mistrusting – the list is almost endless. How do we act and react? For quite some time now, I have been trying to decode the messages conveyed to me through other people for myself. How am I? How do I behave? What impression do I make on others? In doing this, I get to know myself better and have the opportunity to change. Sometimes we are afraid of other people and their reactions, which is why we let ourselves be manipulated and exploited. Or, by being on "good behaviour" and serving others, we want to make them love us.

Mudras 1, 12, 14, 45, and 47 can bring clarity into our relationships, take away fear, and support the work of forgiveness. However, at this point I would like to ask a great favour of you. If, with all of this self-contemplation, you notice how you still do things "wrong" time and time again, love yourself and pamper yourself. And, in particular, laugh about yourself instead of criticising and scolding. There is always the next time to try and "do things right." I'll keep my fingers crossed for you.

Mudras for Solving Everyday Problems

Common sense tells us that every problem contains its own solution. It is part of human nature to be repeatedly faced with challenges, situations, and problems that demand a solution. This keeps us alert, sharpens our senses, and challenges our rational mind. In the silence of meditation we can go into our depths and come into contact with the Highest. Here we can ask, and the right answer always comes in the right way through another person, a book, a voice on the radio, a feeling, or in some other way, and at the right time. I could tell you lots interesting stories on this theme that I learned while seeking the wisdom of the mudras. This is almost a wonder! My husband recently remarked, "You are either the luckiest person on Earth or a witch!" But, obviously, neither of these are true. I have attained a good portion of confidence and trust in the cosmic forces because of all my experiences – that is my luck today. But it wasn't always that way!

When making decisions, whether they are small or large, never forget to make use of meditation. And if there is something that you absolutely want to have, but don't receive it (when an apartment or a job gets taken away from under your nose, etc.), then there is certain to be something better waiting for you.

The following mudras are particularly suited for solving everyday problems: 14, 16, 18, 31, 42, 50, and 51.

Mudras for Building Character

We all have character traits that make life difficult or uncomfortable for us (exaggerated fearfulness, being overly critical, feelings of guilt, addictive behaviour, inferiority complexes, nervousness, pessimism, etc.). Meditation is a wonderful way to transform or even completely reverse them. The best approach is to just deal with one at a time. If we are successful in changing just one single character trait a year, then how will we be in ten years? We shouldn't fight against a character trait that we want to get rid of; instead, we should scrutinise it and even recognise its good aspects. This is the only way that we can let go of it.

First ask yourself where this unattractive trait comes from, how it developed, what is good about it (there is something good in everything). Each uncomfortable trait can show you the way to something better. Unfortunately, you can also be defeated because of one. Or you can become stronger. Then get a very detailed, clear image of the benefits of changing the character trait into its opposite. Now you can decide whether to live with it in peace, by placing limitations on it, or get rid of it by imagining situations in which you live with the opposite trait (for example, courage instead of fear). Your inner images will gradually move into the outside world and become your outer reality.

We can include all these considerations in meditation (Mudras 13, 22, 23, 24, 30, and 38). Then we will experience true wonders.

Mudras for Planning the Future

How many people are afraid of the future, afraid of losing their jobs, of getting old, of all the possible diseases? I once asked a large group about fear of the future. Everyone was surprised about the variety of fears that came to light. The human imagination knows no boundaries here! Some people had fears that seemed totally unimaginable to the others. Everyone agreed at the conclusion – there is hardly a human being who takes a "realistic" look at the future.

Why not fundamentally get rid of unnecessary fears right now! Meditation can be used as a way to visualise images of the future, to plan short-term and long-term goals. Most people do this unconsciously anyway, but we can consciously plan a future that we find suitable, enjoyable, and meaningful. Most of my inner plans have become outer reality within twelve years. Some of them are still open, and I know that these will also be fulfiled at the right time. Incidentally, I have made an interesting discovery. People usually die in the way that they imagine they will.

Mudras 2, 8, 16, 18, 24, 32, and 42 are suitable for helping to plan your future.

Mudras for Connecting with the Divine

Have you ever read that a person will be asked at Heaven's gate if he or she has prayed or meditated enough while on Earth? Definitely not. It doesn't matter how *often* we sit or kneel and meditate, but rather *how and whether* we have lived a fulfiled life and expressed the will of cosmic consciousness through what we have done and not done. Our task in life consists of doing our best and leaving the works up to the Divine before and after their completion. The supreme rule of all great religious communities has always been, "Pray and work." We don't have to join an order to do this; we can also do it alone.

Mudras 19, 40, 42, 43, 44, 45, 46, 47, 48, 49, 50, 51, and 52 help us find repose and also lead us to inner peace, contentment, and joy. In turn, we should let peace and joy flow into our words and works, carrying them out into the world.

MEDITATIONS
FOR EACH FINGER

*T*he following meditations will help you consciously experience your individual fingers and the strength within them. You will become acquainted with your fingers, learning to trust and love them. The positive experiences that I have had confirm that the classification of chakra energy with each of the fingers is accurate. It meaningfully complements the meridian system. (You can learn more about chakras in Appendix D.) Your conscious and constructive thoughts are also useful here. As already mentioned, thoughts and feelings influence every body function. What you "set your heart on" and "talk yourself into" will manifest itself within a foreseeable amount of time.

Hindu healing practitioners already discovered long ago that too much or too little of an element (earth, water, air, fire, and ether) causes the body to become imbalanced or even seriously ill. See page 30 for more information on this topic. We can restore the harmony within us through the corresponding images. Just as every element can have a positive influence on us, it can also destroy us. The individual elements naturally influence each other. Every element has special needs that can be easily satisfied in a balanced and calm dynamic state. But how often are we stressed, rest and exercise too little, eat too much, or let ourselves be plagued by worries? All of this throws us off balance. When the body is no longer capable of attaining harmony, we are out of balance and we become susceptible to disease.

The following meditations can be done during the sleepless hours of a long night or an illness. It demands nothing more of the body than lovingly embracing one finger with the fingers of the other hand.

Meditation 1: Thumb Energy

The fire element, the lung meridian, and Mars (the planet and/or ancient god of war) are associated with the thumb. The fire of the thumb nourishes the energy of the other fingers and absorbs excess energy. It thereby restores equilibrium. When we think about the incineration of garbage, we sense that destruction through fire can also have a power that creates order. Even in nature, when during the course of the decades a monoculture of the strongest has been created, the forest fire once again creates the preconditions for a larger variety of new plants. The overheating within our bodies, the fever, kills entire cultures of bacteria. Fire is dependent upon air since it dies without oxygen; the same also applies to our cell respiration. The metabolism in the individual cells can only properly function with adequate oxygen. We can actually strengthen every part of the body or every organ by visualising and/or breathing light and warmth into it.

∼ Exercise ∼

Either sit or lie down. Now encircle your right thumb with the four fingers of your left hand and place your left thumb along the inner edge of your right hand. Close your eyes.

> *Focus on a part of the body that is weak or ill. Now imagine that a light is burning in the lower centre of your body (at the height of the navel). Every time you exhale, direct the rays of light toward the respective part of the body. First let large, dark clouds of smoke*

(things that make you ill, pain, etc.) escape from the illuminated body part. Then concentrate solely on the light that slowly fills, illuminates, and heals this part of the body.

Calmly keep holding onto your thumb for a while and feel the flowing warmth. Then encircle your left thumb and also hold this for a while.

Meditation 2: Index Finger Energy

The heart chakra, the large intestine, and the deep meridian of the stomach are associated with this finger. Here we also find the "sure" instinct, having "a good nose," the ability to reflect, and inspiration. This energy goes to our innermost core and back to the cosmos from there. We can also draw on our innermost being (intuition) and receive from the cosmos (inspiration). This finger includes both closeness and expansiveness. How much closeness can we stand?

The air element represents the mind – the power of thought. Thoughts are as invisible as the air and yet, as the yogis have discovered, they are the cause of all the actions that we take or refrain from taking, of everything that we reject and attract, for our health and for every mood, and for the entire design of our life. The planetary power of Jupiter is also associated with this finger, and indicates the eternal change of things – accepting life with all its facets, working through (digesting), and letting go again.

There is also a clear, purposeful look into the future in this finger. Since our thoughts are so important, we should consider their quality more frequently. If we do the following meditation several days in a row, we will notice that there is a certain habit in our thoughts. Habits can be changed as soon as we become aware of them, but changes always require a certain amount of time. If we continuously replace harmful thoughts with useful ones, we can also change the circumstances of life accordingly.

～ Exercise ～

Sit or lie down. Now encircle your right index finger with the four fingers of your left hand, letting the thumb extend to the middle of your right hand. Close your eyes.

> *You are sitting in front of a field and observe the swaying ears of grain. When you inhale, the ears of grain move toward you. When you exhale, they move away from you. Sometimes you see the entire field, and sometimes you see the individual ears of grain. You also see how the space gets smaller when you inhale, and larger when you exhale. The yellow ears indicate transience, the great dying that is already contained in the seed of a new beginning. After a while, look into the expanse of the blue clouded sky and then inwardly to the safety of your own heart. Now observe the thoughts that come and go, and think about your thoughts for a while. How do you think most of the time? In a positive, negative, confident, fearful, brooding (turning over worries), critical, memory-dominated, or future-oriented way?*

Keep holding onto your finger for a while and feel the flowing warmth. Then encircle your left index finger and also hold this for a while.

Meditation 3: Middle Finger Energy

Hindus call this finger the heavenly finger and classify it with the throat chakra. Take a look at it. It is the longest finger, and towers over the others. Its energy radiates far into infinity. It could also be considered the stairway to Heaven. Saturn, which is classified with it, is located toward the edge of our solar system and is also called the "keeper of the threshold." We are held accountable for our lives at the gates of Heaven. We also find this symbolism in the throat chakra, the gateway of purity, which only opens when the student is pure in spirit and in heart. However, in order to progress on our spiritual path, we must first fulfil our duties on Earth. This is indicated by its inherent meridians: the circulation meridian and the deep meridian of the gallbladder. Both help us seize and master the challenges of life. Drive, activity, risk, and the joy of taking action are their qualities. The spectrum of the middle-finger energy ranges from an active life to spheres far into the world beyond. It could be briefly summarised with the following saying, "God helps those who help themselves."

∿ Exercise ∿

Sit or lie down. Now encircle your right middle finger with the four fingers of your left hand. The left thumb extends to the middle of your right hand. Close your eyes.

> *Imagine yourself doing what you like to do most. Make full use of your inclinations and talents as you master all the obstacles placed in your path, and enjoy your activities. You are successful at what you do and mentally envision what your success looks like. What you do enriches the world (your family, individual human beings, or the entire world). Extensively imagine the constant contact with the divine forces that help you and show you the way.*

> *If your occupation does not satisfy you and if you have no leisure activities or interests that suit you, then it is time to ask within, to press your inner wisdom until you receive an answer. At the same time, also ask for the initiative, which the middle finger symbolises, to actually tackle the matter at hand. And, above all, request help from the divine powers – enter into a close, trusting partnership with them.*

Keep holding your finger in silence for a while and feel the warmth flowing

into you. Then encircle your left middle finger and hold it for a while.
These hand positions also have an excellent effect on tension in the neck.

Meditation 4: Ring Finger Energy

The ring finger is associated with Apollo, the sun god, and the root chakra,
which rules the pelvic floor. This force gives stamina, staying power, and
the power to be assertive. The Chinese have classified this finger with the
deep meridian of the liver. The power of the liver gives a person patience,
serenity, hope, and vision for the future. The "triple warmer" also begins
in the tip of the ring finger. This meridian rules all protective functions in
the body and is responsible for body temperature, which in turn regulates
cell function. If it works in an optimal manner, it gives the ability to maintain our equilibrium in stressful situations, which is also the precondition
for a well-functioning immune system. The force that dominates this finger provides stability, is penetrating, and strives upward.

∽ Exercise ∽

Sit or lie down. Now encircle your left ring finger with the four fingers of
your right hand, with the right thumb extending to the middle of your left
hand. Close your eyes.

Imagine bare earth and crushed rock in all its forms – as deserts,
mountains, and islands. What happens when masses of earth begin
to move? When the earth dries out? When the earth is completely
exposed to the sun? Now imagine fertile earth. Slowly let the vege-
tation be created – little plants, big plants, much green. Now focus
on one single seed resting deep within the earth. With every breath,
something moves inside until the seed bursts and a shoot stretches in

the direction of the light. At the same time, it sprouts roots deep into the earth. It becomes a tree that grows very slowly. You wait patiently and watch how the plant develops into its full size. Time has no significance. Only the constant growth counts. The tree blooms anew every year, and bears fruit. Like the tree, we also do not know why this is. Like the tree, we want to give ourselves completely to life, and know this has its purpose, even if we will probably never be able to completely fathom the great mystery. As the tree changes every year, our inner development also continues. We decisively influence whether it is joyful or sorrowful.

Keep holding your finger for a while and feel the flowing warmth. Then encircle your right ring finger and hold it for the same amount of time.

Meditation 5: Little Finger Energy

The second chakra, which is the energetic centre of sexuality, is associated with the little finger. It deals with interpersonal relationships in general, as well as partnership in particular. This classification of sexuality corresponds with Hatha Yoga. (In Buddhism, sexuality is associated with the ring finger.) It also contains the ability to communicate. Since the Chinese healing practitioners found the heart meridian to be in this finger, this confirms the yogis' thesis relating the water element to it (water symbolises the realm of the emotions). Joyful, fulfiling relationships not only warm the heart, but also nourish and strengthen it. And, in turn, strong heart energy gives us the ability to be happy. It gives us sublime feelings and improves our mood. Our mood, which is always the sum of present feelings, can be compared with the waves on the surface of a lake. They are rhythmically harmonious or vehement; the water is clear and clean, or shallow, heavy, dark and dirty.

∾ Exercise ∾

Sit or lie down. Now encircle your left little finger with the four fingers of your right hand, with your right thumb extending to the middle of your left hand. Close your eyes.

In your mind's eye, you are sitting by the sea and observing the waves – they come toward you, and roll back out and disappear. The same applies to your feelings, moods, and also to your relationships with others. Giving and receiving love is also subject to this law. Be aware that you only receive as much love as you can unconditionally give. This doesn't even have to mean great deeds. A friendly, warm heart for fellow human beings, animals, plants, water, air, and earth are entirely enough. Imagine someone (someone specific or in general) happy and encourage him or her, if necessary. Believe in this individual's abilities and good heart. Imagine entire scenes in which this person is cheerful and smiling happily. If you have no one close to you, then do this little exercise – perhaps while riding the bus, train, or streetcar – in relation to a stranger. I guarantee that you will experience wonders if you keep this up for several days or weeks. The time will come when your heart will overflow with joy. But the most important thing is: don't expect anything at all for the time being. Radiate your goodwill and your love unconditionally. Just have some patience until the seeds sprout.

Continue holding your little finger for a while and feel the flowing warmth. Then encircle your right little finger and hold it for the same amount of time.

PART TWO

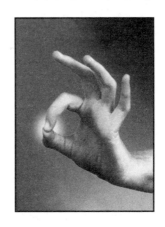

The

Mudras

MUDRAS FOR THE BODY, MIND, AND SOUL

*T*he following mudras are primarily used to support the healing or relief of physical complaints. Combined with visualisations and affirmations, they also influence our minds and emotional responses to life.

As I mentioned earlier, no health disorder comes out of the blue. If we meditate and use the mudras to simply get rid of symptoms of illness or pain, we are burying our heads in the sand. There may be short-term results, but not lasting healing. The best thing to do is to use the mudras, plants, and other healing remedies for our healing, while we simultaneously examine why we feel this way in the first place. *First:* what is the true cause? During meditation, we can ask our inner wisdom, our higher self, or the divine light about the cause of an illness. Perhaps the cause is quite easy to find. We simply ate the wrong thing or were stressed; or we didn't rest enough and our immune system is stressed. Negative feelings, such as resentment, hate, revenge, envy, and miserliness, also make us sick. Particularly in the case of chronic health disorders, negative feelings are frequently the cause. *Second:* what "advantages of illness" does the disease give me? There is an advantage in every illness – finally getting enough rest, other people looking after us, sympathy, being able to pass on responsibility, and so on. We must also allow ourselves to have affection, sympathy, and rest in the proper proportions and not expect it from others. We can change a few habits so that we get the "advantages of illness" without being sick.

Third: we must be willing to let go of everything that makes us ill. The shamans of native peoples always drive off the evil spirits at the beginning of their healing rituals. Consider what (or who makes you sick. Which thoughts, feelings, and habits undermine your health? Are you willing to give them up? This self-analysis, the research into why I become ill, has given my life a completely new quality; but it did demand quite a bit of honesty from me. Moreover, looking at yourself isn't a closed chapter, but a continuous path of self-knowledge. Yet, despite the honesty and rigorousness, please don't forget love, loving care, and understanding for yourself. The more you fail, the more you need your own love.

1

GANESHA MUDRA

(The elephant; Ganesha, the deity who overcomes all obstacles)

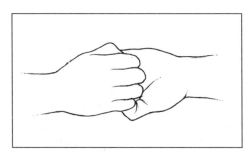

Hold your left hand in front of your chest with the palm facing outward. Bend the fingers. Now grasp the left hand with the right hand, which has its back facing outward. Move the hands to the level of the heart, right in front of the chest. While exhaling, vigorously pull the hands apart without releasing the grip. This will tense the muscles of the upper arms and chest area. While inhaling, let go of all the tension. Repeat 6 times and then lovingly place both hands on the sternum in this position. Focus on the feeling in this part of your body. Then change the hand position: your right palm now faces outward. Repeat the exercise 6 times in this position. Afterward, remain in silence for a while.

Once a day is enough.

VARIATION: Repeat the same exercise, but this time keep the lower arms diagonal instead of horizontal: one elbow points upward at a slant and the other elbow points downward at a slant.

This mudra stimulates heart activity, strengthens heart muscles, opens the bronchial tubes, and releases any type of tension in this area. It opens the fourth chakra and gives us courage, confidence, and openness toward other human beings.

I find it interesting that I make precisely this gesture when I want to encourage another person, "Muster up your courage – seize the opportunity – you can do it!" It is as if the hands strengthen the words, and the heart as well. The famous "jungle doctor" Albert Schweitzer addressed the problem on another level when he said that many people appear to be "cold" because they cannot risk showing themselves to be as warmhearted as they are.

HERBAL REMEDY: Hawthorn (*Crataegus oxyacantha L.*) strengthens the heart.

Since the Ganesha Mudra activates the fire element (see Appendix C), which reacts positively to the colour red, the following visualisations support activity of the heart and circulation. It encourages us to encounter our fellow human beings with an open and friendly heart.

Visualise the colour red – a mosaic, a mandala, or a carpet in various tones of red. Now focus all of your senses on it for a while. Red should strengthen, warm, and widen your heart, giving you the courage to be open and confident.

Affirmation
I meet other people with courage, openness, and confidence.

2

USHAS MUDRA

(Break of day – origin of all good things)

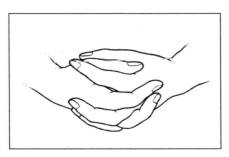

Clasp your fingers so your right thumb lies above the left. The right thumb presses slightly on the left thumb.

Important: Women should place the right thumb between the left thumb and index finger, pressing on it with the left thumb.

Do this every day for 5 to 15 minutes. Hold this mudra until the desired effect occurs.

No matter how old we are, there are times of change: new beginnings come repeatedly in life. The second chakra, our centre of sexuality and creativity, always contains something new, a secret that wants to be aired. This mudra concentrates the sexual energy of our second chakra and directs it into the energy centres above it. It gives us mental alertness, pleasure, and new impulses. In addition, it harmonises our hormonal system.

The Ushas Mudra helps us wake up in the morning. When you are still sleepy and lying in bed, place your clasped hands at the back of your head. Now inhale vigorously and deeply several times; open your eyes and mouth widely; press your elbows back into the pillow. While exhaling, let go of every tension. Repeat 6 times. If this still doesn't make you feel alert and fresh, then rub your ankle bones together, as well as the palms of your hands, as if you were trying to ignite a flintstone. Finally, you can also extend your arms and stretch vigorously, as shown on page 63.

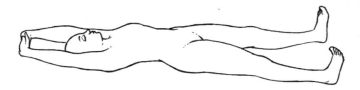

HERBAL REMEDY: Green tea and rosemary *(Rosmarinus officinalis L.)* have a refreshing effect.

In your imagination, see yourself sitting in a good place where you can enjoy the sunrise. The sun slowly rises, and you let the colours red, orange, and yellow have their effect on you for a long time. These colours awaken and improve your mood. Now imagine yourself as a person who is full of youthful strength and new impulses, as someone who enjoys life, a person who goes out into the world with love, and richly blesses it with a sincere smile, good deeds, and beautiful things.

Affirmation
I am filled with pleasure and enthusiasm, which allow me to achieve great things. I enjoy life to the fullest.

3

PUSHAN MUDRA

(Dedicated to the sun god, Pushan, also the god of nourishment)

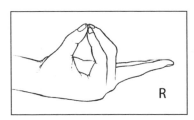

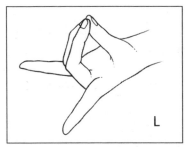

VERSION 1:

Right hand: The tips of the thumb, index finger, and middle finger are on top of each other; the other fingers are extended.

Left hand: The tips of the thumb, middle finger, and ring finger are on top of each other; the other fingers are extended.

This mudra symbolises accepting and receiving with the gesture of one hand and letting things flow, giving, and letting go with the gesture of the other. Both should be coordinated with each other in digestion. It influences the energy currents that are responsible for absorbing and utilising food, as well as helping with elimination. It intensifies breathing and therefore the absorption of oxygen and the release of carbon dioxide in the lungs. It has a relaxing effect on the solar plexus (the area of the stomach, liver, spleen, and gallbladder), regulates energies in the autonomic nervous system, mobilises energies of elimination, and detoxifies. It has an excellent effect on general or acute nausea, seasickness, flatulence, and that sensation of fullness one feels after meals.

VERSION 2:

Right hand: The tips of the thumb, ring finger, and little finger are on top of each other, the other fingers are extended.

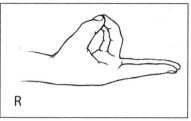

Left hand: Same as Version 1.
Connecting the energies of the thumb, ring finger, and little finger activates the lower digestive process and the elimination process. This mudra can be called the general energy pump. It stimulates the functions of the brain, a fact that has also been proved scientifically. The finger position of the right hand activates energy in the pelvic floor, like a smoldering fire that has been stoked. With the finger position of the left hand, the kindled energy is directed upward. Every organ, the general mood, and thinking (concentration, memory, logic, enthusiasm, etc.) are positively influenced as a result.

These two mudras can be used as immediate help or practised four times a day for 5 minutes in the case of chronic complaints.

HERBAL REMEDY: Fennel *(Foeniculum vulgare), anise (Pimpinella anisum),* and caraway *(Carum carvi)* support this mudra.

During *inhalation,* take in energy in the form of light. During the pause in breathing, give it the time and space it needs to spread within you and become transformed. During *exhalation,* let the expended energy flow back out of you. With every breath, there is more light and clarity in your physical and mental-emotional realms.

Affirmation
I thankfully accept everything that is good for me, let it have its effect within me, and release everything that is spent.

BRONCHIAL MUDRA

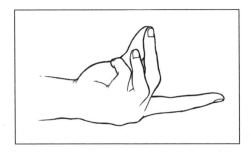

Both hands: Place the little finger at the base of the thumb, the ring finger on the upper thumb joint, and the middle finger on the pad of the thumb. Extend the index finger.

For an acute attack of asthma, first use this mudra from 4 to 6 minutes and then practise the Asthma Mudra (Number 5) until breathing has become normal again. For a long-term treatment, hold both mudras for 5 minutes, five times a day.

People with respiratory problems often also suffer from inner loneliness, isolation, sexual problems, and sadness. To the outside world, these feelings are often successfully played down with humour. Or these individuals bind themselves to others by taking on their duties and concerns. This naturally causes a great deal of stress so that these individuals are pressed for time and out of breath. Since I am all too familiar with such problems, I can perhaps advise you how to get out of this dilemma. It is important to admit your negative feelings and moods for once and take a good look at them. Be aware that even these feelings are like waves on the surface of the water – they arise and then pass on. The reason for such feelings is often a general weakness that is caused by shallow breathing since improper respiration doesn't build up the inner reservoir of strength. When it is reduced, weakness occurs not only on the physical level but also in the mental-emotional area. Fear, sadness, discontentment, exaggerated sensitivity, etc., are the consequences.

In yoga, *every* breathing exercise and physical exercise builds up this inner strength and keeps up the energy level (practise for at least 30 minutes every day – you can find the appropriate sequence of exercises on pages 177–189). The following mudra meditation is also effective. Sit upright and hold your hands about 4 inches away from your body. When your arms get tired, place the hands on your thighs.

HERBAL REMEDY: Thyme *(Thymus serpyllum L.), primrose (Primula veris L.),* and elder *(Sambucus nigra L.)* are the most important herbs for the bronchial tubes.

Direct your consciousness to the pelvic floor and sense the surface you are sitting on. *Inhalation:* Now direct your consciousness into your abdomen, stomach, chest, throat, forehead, and top of the head. Count from 1 to 7 while you do so. Now hold your breath for about 5 seconds. *Exhalation:* Direct your consciousness from top to bottom and count backward from 7 to 1. Wait patiently until the impulse to inhale comes, and then direct the consciousness back to the top again while inhaling. *The pauses after inhaling and exhaling are very important here.*

Affirmation
*Every breath gives me strength. It strengthens my
body, mind, and soul.*

5

ASTHMA MUDRA

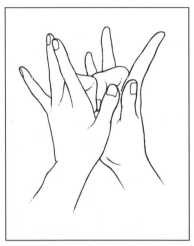

Both hands: Press together the finger-nails of the middle fingers and keep other fingers extended.

In case of an acute asthma attack, first do the Bronchial Mudra (Number 4) for 4 to 6 minutes. Then use this Asthma Mudra until the breathing calms down. For long-term treatment, use these two mudras five times every day for 5 minutes.

Unfortunately, I am not one of those fortunate people who once had asthma but got rid of it through a radical cure with medication and never felt anything again. Many members of my family on my father's side had asthma, so it is a "dear" family heirloom. But despite this, I live without any medication because I follow certain rules of behaviour. My tips are sure to help asthma patients, which is why I'm passing them on here:

- During cold weather, never breathe through your mouth because the bronchial tubes will become inflamed and congested.
- Try not to be in a hurry because every incidence of stress activates the adrenal glands. Adrenaline promotes the congestion and constriction of the bronchial tubes.
- Eat a light diet with little meat; meat once a week is enough.

No milk products, tomatoes, hot peppers, or kiwi. No smoking should be obvious.

- Don't take medications that weaken the immune system, such as antibiotics.
- Get enough fresh air by taking long walks. Do yoga or gymnastics every week and get enough rest.

Most people who suffer from breathing difficulties are familiar with inner loneliness (too much detachment from the surrounding world) and/or cannot set boundaries. Consequently, they feel themselves plagued by other people's duties and problems (too little detachment).

HERBAL REMEDY: Horehound *(Marrubium vulgare L.)* and black cumin *(Nigella sativa)* help against asthma complaints.

Visualise pictures of a wide expanse – the ocean, the sky with clouds, and mountains (you stand on the peak). Take this expansiveness into your heart and lung area. While *exhaling,* let the distances become greater; while *inhaling,* let them become smaller again – a proportion that is right for you. Now do the same with the people or duties that you find oppressive.

Affirmation
I detach myself from everything that constricts me and fully enjoy my new freedom. I feel safe and secure in the divine light, which gives me support.

PRAN MUDRA

(Life Mudra)

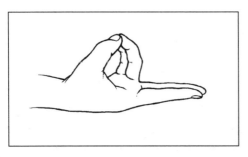

With each hand: Place the tips of the thumb, ring finger, and little finger together. The other fingers remain extended.

As needed, use for 5 to 30 minutes. Or, as a course of treatment, do three times a day for 15 minutes.

The Pran Mudra activates the root chakra (see Appendix D), in which the elemental force of a human being is found. I like to compare this place with a fire that is either ablaze or just glows quietly. How brightly the fire burns depends on how well we tend it. This finger position stimulates the nourishing energy in the pelvic floor.

The Pran Mudra generally increases vitality, reduces fatigue and nervousness, and improves vision. It is also used against eye diseases. On the mental-emotional level, it increases our staying power and assertiveness, healthy self-confidence, gives us the courage to start something new, and the strength to see things through. Clear eyes are also a sign of a mental outlook emphasising clarity and a clear mind, which means clearly structured thoughts and ideas.

According to Kim da Silva, when you do the Pran Mudra you can also put your thumb onto the fingernails of the other two fingers instead of on their tips. This has the effect of causing both the right and left brain hemispheres to function equally, become active, and mutually complement each other, which is very important for holistic health.

Nervousness is usually a sign of weakness, of too much distraction and too little inner stability. The Pran Mudra – combined with a conscious, slow, and gentle way of breathing – has the effect of being as stabilising and calming as a secure anchor.

HERBAL REMEDY: Passionflower *(Passiflora caerulea L.)*, St. John's wort *(Hypericum perforatum L.)*, and oat *(Avena sativa L.)* strengthen the nervous system and support staying power.

Imagine yourself as a tree. If this is difficult for you, then create the mental image of a tree in front of you. While *inhaling,* see how the energy flows into the roots and how the roots become thicker and longer. While *exhaling,* let the strength flow into the trunk. From there, it travels into the crown, far beyond the tree into the sky and toward the sun. The larger the rootstock becomes, the greater the size of the crown. The same also applies to us, to our existence, how we act, and what we have.

Affirmation
I have a healthy appetite for the small and large adventures of life. I digest the challenges with great pleasure and joy.

7

LINGA MUDRA

(Upright Mudra)

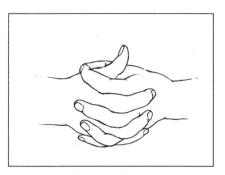

Place both palms together and clasp your fingers. One thumb should remain upright; encircle it with the thumb and index finger of your other hand.

Do as needed or three times a day for 15 minutes.

This finger position increases the powers of resistance against coughs, colds, and chest infections. It also loosens mucus that has collected in the lungs. In addition, it is very useful for people who suffer from respiratory complaints when the weather changes. It also increases the body temperature and is particularly suited for people who don't develop a fever that is high enough. Fever is important because many bacteria within the body can only be killed when it reaches a certain temperature.

The Linga Mudra can, according to Keshav Dev, also help reduce weight. However, for this purpose it must be done with particular care three times a day for 15 minutes. Also drink at least 8 glasses of water a day, and mainly eat cooling foods, such as yogurt, rice, bananas, and citrus fruits. If the Linga Mudra is done too long, a feeling of sluggishness and lethargy may occur. This is a sign that you should shorten the length of this exercise and consume more cooling foods and drinks.

In order to stimulate your immune system and increase body temperature, you can practise the following exercise before doing the Linga

Mudra. It is appropriately called "Throwing the Illness Behind You." Then do the Linga Mudra while sitting or lying down until you feel very hot.

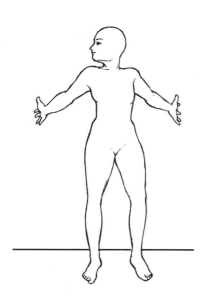

Basic position: Stand up; legs are slightly spread, knees bent somewhat, and hands are in front of the chest.

Inhalation: Throw your arms behind you, turn your head to the right, and look over your shoulder.

Exhalation: Return your hands to your chest and turn your head to the front.

Repeat at least ten times.

HERBAL REMEDY: Echinacea *(Echinacea angustifolia)* is generally recommended for activation of the immune system.

Imagine a fire within your body that burns the bacteria, waste, and unnecessary ballast.

Affirmation
My powers of resistance develop more and more
from moment to moment.

8

APAN MUDRA

(Energy Mudra)

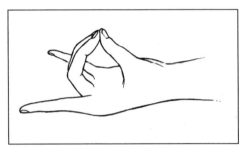

With each hand: Place the thumb, middle finger, and ring finger together – extend the other fingers.

When needed, do for 5 to 45 minutes or use three times a day for 15 minutes as a course of treatment.

This mudra supports the removal of waste materials and toxins from the body, as well as eliminating urinary problems, according to Keshav Dev.

The Apan Mudra also stimulates the wood element, which is associated with the energy of the liver and gallbladder (see Appendix C). This element also contains the power and pleasure of springtime, of new beginnings, of tackling and shaping visions of the future.

In addition, the Apan Mudra has a balancing effect on the mind, which is largely dependent upon a well-functioning liver. It gives us patience, serenity, confidence, inner balance, and harmony. In the mental realm, it creates the ability to develop vision. You need all of this when you look into the future, while facing new challenges, and if your wishes are to be fulfiled.

HERBAL REMEDY: Two wonder remedies for the liver and gallbladder are milk thistle *(Silybum marianum)* and dandelion *(Taraxacum officinale)*.

In your imagination, sit in a beautiful, richly blossoming garden. You enjoy the various colours and forms of the plants. You observe the great mystery of nature – how a seed germinates, how a plant grows and blooms. Now, in an empty bed, plant something that should bear rich fruits for you: a conversation, a relationship, a project, etc. Imagine how it sprouts, continues to develop, blossoms, and bears rich fruit. Who should benefit from these fruits? End this image with a big thank you.

Affirmation
I plant my seeds, care for them, and receive a rich harvest –
with God's help – that I thankfully accept.

9

SHANKH MUDRA

(Shell Mudra)

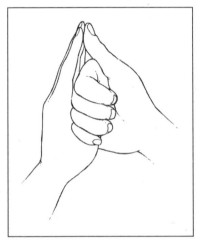

Encircle the your thumb with the four fingers of your right hand. At the same time, touch the right thumb to the extended middle finger of your left hand. Together, the two hands look like a conch shell. Hold your hands in front of your sternum.

Do this as often and as long as you want. Or use it three times daily for 15 minutes as a course of treatment.

When you want to practise this mudra, you can first sing "OM" several times. Then listen within yourself, to the silence, for several minutes afterward.

This mudra is used during rituals in many Hindu temples. There, the conch horn is blown in the morning to announce the opening of the temple doors. The same applies to our inner temple, in which the divine light shines – it should also be opened.

The Shell Mudra drives away every kind of problem in the throat. If you practise it regularly, especially if you sing "OM" as you do it, you can improve your voice. It also has a very calming effect and leads to collection in silence.

HERBAL REMEDY: If you have throat problems, it helps to gargle with sage tea that has a few drops of lemon juice and some honey added to it.

First let yourself be brought into collected repose through the mudra and by singing OM. See your hands as a seashell and the encircled thumb as the pearl within it. Your left thumb becomes the symbol of the higher self, with which you connect yourself in love, and which lets you receive all the help you require, or which gives you confidence and a sense of security – simply everything you need.

Affirmation
I use thoughts and words of strength and love, and everything that I think and speak comes back to me.

10

SURABHI MUDRA

(Cow Mudra)

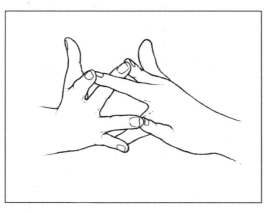

The little finger of your left hand touches the ring finger of your right hand. The little finger of your right hand touches the ring finger of your left hand. At the same time, the middle fingers of both hands touch the index fingers of the other. The thumbs remain extended.

Do three times a day for 15 minutes.

The Surabhi Mudra is very effective against rheumatism and arthrosis. Since these diseases are usually chronic, or at least have existed within the person long before any outbreak or pain is perceived, this mudra must also be practised for a longer period of time.

HERBAL REMEDY: A person with these complaints should also be sure to eat a healthy and light diet (see Appendix A) and drink a great deal of green tea. In addition, rampion *(Harpagophytum procumbens DC)* can be used to put an end to annoying rheumatism and arthrosis.

At first, mainly concentrate on your exhalation and imagine how a dark cloud leaves your body each time you *exhale.* This cloud contains your spent energy, all the waste substances, and every pain. Most importantly, it also contains all your negative thoughts and feelings. After about 20 breaths, also pay attention to your *inhalation,* and imagine each time that you are absorbing light, which makes your entire body shine. Gradually let the cloud that you exhale become lighter and lighter. In conclusion, let yourself be filled with the brightest light and surrounded by a cloak of light that radiates far out into your environment.

Affirmation

Purifying light fills me and burns away everything that oppresses and hurts me. From the bottom of my heart, I seek cleanliness in my body, clarity in my mind, and purity in my soul.

11

VAYU MUDRA

(Wind Mudra)

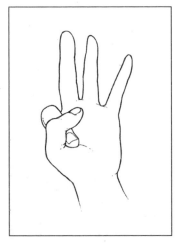

With each hand bend the index finger so that its tip touches the ball of the thumb. Then press the thumb lightly onto the index finger. Extend the other fingers in a relaxed way.

For chronic complaints, do this mudra three times daily for 15 minutes; otherwise, use it until it has an effect.

This position prevents "wind" (meaning flatulence), and a sensation of fullness, in all parts of the body. Ayurvedic medicine assumes that there are 51 types of wind in the body that produce numerous disorders. These include gout, sciatica, flatulence, rheumatism, and trembling in the hands, throat, and head. If you use the Vayu Mudra within 24 hours after an outbreak of a disorder or disease caused by wind, you can very quickly count on improvement. For chronic complaints, the Pran Mudra (Number 6) on page 70 should be practised. The Vayu Mudra must be discontinued as soon as the disease disappears.

Too much wind in the body can be caused by inner waste substances, particularly in the intestines, or inner tensions that are in turn based on states of agitation. Frequently, the normal breathing rhythm (which is different for each individual) is also disrupted.

As an additional measure, the "stomach contractor" can also be practised. To do this, assume the "cat posture." *Inhale* and lift your head some-

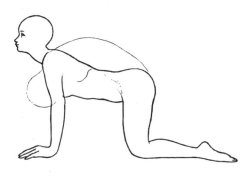

what; *exhale* and lower your head again while vigorously pulling in the abdominal wall at the same time. During the pause in breathing, pull in the abdominal wall and let go of it several times. Then inhale deeply again; raise your head again. Repeat the whole exercise a number of times.

In addition, the following visualisation can help against tensions and states of agitation.

Imagine that you are standing in a storm. While exhaling, blow out all your inner tensions and waste substances into the wind. Now the storm is dying down and you also become calm by letting your exhalation become slower and more calm again. Now lengthen the pauses between inhalation and exhalation. The air has a fine texture as it streams into your lungs; slowly and peacefully it leaves you again. Let yourself sink into a pleasant state of relaxation, from which new strength can develop.

Affirmation
I am calm and serene at any time and in any place.

12

SHUNYA MUDRA

(Heaven Mudra)

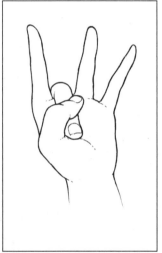

Bend the middle finger until it touches the ball of your thumb. Lightly press down on the middle finger with your thumb. The other fingers are extended. Do this with each hand.

Do as needed, or use three times daily for 15 minutes as a course of treatment.

This is a special exercise against ear and hearing problems. The Shunya Mudra can also quickly heal earaches (and almost all diseases of the ear) when used for a longer period of time, according to Keshav Dev.

Hearing problems are related to a person who is no longer able to hear or who even doesn't want to hear. This can be a blessing or a catastrophe. Poor hearing can protect us from unpleasant things or even from disagreeable sounds or information that find their way into us. On the other hand, we can also no longer hear beautiful things. Not wanting to hear is sometimes based on a particular kind of stubbornness that can lead to disaster. Consequently, if we are willing to scrutinise the reason for our hearing problems, this can lead us one step further toward a richer life.

The middle finger is associated with the sky (ether). This is the gateway to the higher dimensions – the gateway to Heaven. The ancient myths say, if we want to get to Heaven, we first need to be thoroughly purified.

This is why it may be appropriate to "look within" and make amends for old offences. I know that it can sometimes be very difficult to forgive another person; but I also know that forgiveness truly opens up new gateways – gateways that lead into the light and into a lightness of the life ahead of us. It is as if we have thrown off our old burdens and then continued happily on our path.

HERBAL REMEDY: A geranium leaf can be placed on a painful ear to soothe it.

Consciously listen to gentle, flowing, and relaxing music. Let thoughts and inner images arise – immediately let go of anything unpleasant – continue imagining pleasant thoughts in keeping with your mood.

Affirmation
I recognise the goodness of the universe in the heavenly sound.

13

PRITHIVI MUDRA

(Earth Mudra)

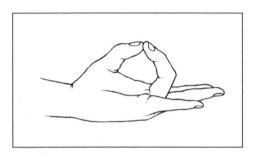

Place the tips of the thumb and ring finger on top of each other, using light pressure. Extend the other fingers. Do this with each hand.

Do as needed, or use three times a day for 15 minutes.

The Prithivi Mudra can eliminate an energy deficit in the root chakra. Whether or not you feel psychologically or physically strong and vital is largely dependent upon this energy. This finger position also intensifies the sense of smell and is good for the nails, skin, hair, and bones. If you feel uncertain of your steps while walking, the Prithivi Mudra can restore your equilibrium and trust. This mudra also activates the root chakra, in which our elemental force resides. We can compare this chakra to the grafting knot of a rose. The potential for the appearance and nature of the plant is found here; the roots sprout into the ground from this point to give the plant stability and absorb the nutrients. The stem and leaves grow upward from this point to connect with the light, to blossom and bear fruit. Without reservation, this image can be applied to human beings as well. We also need stability and nourishment to grow and be effective in our place in the world. The purpose of our lives is to connect with the Divine, which means we must also orient ourselves toward the light and open up like a flower that is being pollinated. For us, this may mean experiencing grace. So this mudra can give us everything that we need for a meaningful life. I use it when I feel insecure and need inner stability and self-assurance. Moreover, it stimulates the body temperature, the liver, and the stomach.

Stand or sit on a chair. Keep your feet parallel and their soles flat on the ground. *Inhalation:* Imagine that you are absorbing Earth energy through the soles of your feet. Guide it up through your legs, back, and throat into your head and far beyond into the cosmos. Hold your breath for a few seconds. *Exhalation:* Like a golden rain, the energy sinks back to Earth as the renewing force. There is a balance between taking and giving. Now imagine a catch basin in your pelvic floor and let the energy rain flow into your pelvis. Repeat this a number of times.

Affirmation
The power of Earth gives me secure stability, staying power and assertiveness, self-assurance, and self-confidence. The power of the cosmos gives me enthusiasm, pleasure, and joy.

14

VARUNA MUDRA

(Varuna is the god of water)

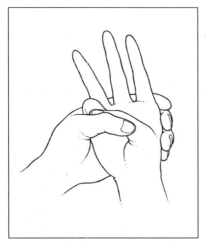

Bend the little finger of your right hand until the tip touches the ball of your right thumb; place the thumb of your right hand on it. Press the little finger and thumb slightly with your left thumb. At the same time, your left hand encircles the right hand lightly from below.

Do as needed, or practise three times a day for 45 minutes.

Keshav Dev says that the Varuna Mudra should always be done when too much mucus or secretion collects in the stomach or lungs. Congestion can settle in the frontal sinuses, lungs, and the entire digestive tract from the stomach to the large intestine. Most allergic reactions are ultimately mucous congestion triggered by specific irritating substances. When we catch a cold, we are usually in a rut in other ways as well. I find this to be 100 percent true for myself. Since I have recognised this fact, I can also do something to relieve the situation (I reduce my workload and my obligations). Mucous congestion, no matter where it occurs in the body, is always related to overstimulated nerves, inner tensions and unrest, triggered by overstraining, being pressed for time, being aggravated, or experiencing fear.

In addition to practicing the Varuna Mudra, it is always important to make a new life plan. Including other people in it is usually good! Perhaps you should rethink your tasks and obligations and reassign some of them to your partner, your child, and/or your parents. People who suffer from mucous congestion are often too conscious of responsibility and think that everything depends on them or that they must do everything alone.

HERBAL REMEDY: A natural remedy against mucous congestion is horseradish, which you can also eat as salad.

The inner image of flowing, lukewarm water that washes away all obligations can be very liberating. Letting everything that burdens you go "down the drain" can give you a wonderful feeling. Imagine that you are standing under a small waterfall. Let everything that sticks to you, both inside and outside, be washed away by the water. Watch how the brown water flows away from you and enjoy your new clean-ness – inner freedom and lightness. Now think about your tasks for a while. At what point can you change something? Where can you reduce your workload? Where can you seek help?

Affirmation
I always have "possibilities" – letting go of something, searching for a solution, and changing things.

15

BHUDI MUDRA

(Fluid Mudra)

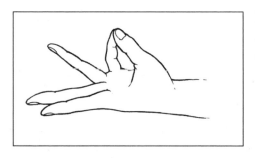

Place the tip of your thumb and little finger together; extend the other fingers in a relaxed way. Do this with each hand.

Do as needed, or practise three times a day for 15 minutes as a course of treatment.

More than half our body weight consists of fluids. The Bhudi Mudra helps restore or maintain equilibrium in the fluid balance. It can be used against a dry mouth, eyes that are too dry and burning, or disorders in the kidney and bladder area. It also improves the sense of taste.

HERBAL REMEDY: Bearberry *(Arctostaphylos uva-ursi L.)* heals inflammation of the bladder, and goldenrod *(Solidasgo virgaurea L.)* is effective against pyelitis.

Even physicians have greatly varying opinions when it comes to how much a person should drink every day. It certainly isn't good to drink too little, but we also don't feel well when we drink too much (even if it is just water). I feel good when I drink about 1 to 1½ quarts of liquid every day. For some time now, I have been drinking water in a way that is connected to a ritual and this has been particularly good for me. My ritual is as follows:

First (blessing water): According to ancient custom, water used for a specific purpose had a spell cast on it, or was blessed. More recent research has discovered that water can actually absorb and store the energy of thoughts and words.

Second (charging water): Water can be either weakly or intensely charged with energy. It depends on the movement that arises when it flows. In a natural stream, where the water is guided from side to side by the stones (and not straight ahead as in a pipe), the energy level is considerably higher. This is why I always stir the water in a glass in the form of an eight for a while.

Third (linking water to the Divine) and probably most important: I consciously connect myself with the Divine, and take in its element with reverence and gratitude. Before I drink the water, I take the glass in both hands in front of my chest, speak my affirmation, and then remain in silence for a few moments. If you drink tap water, please inquire locally about the quality of your water.

Imagine a clear little mountain stream cheerfully splashing as it flows. Dip your feet or hands into it and let it caress you. Draw the water in the hollow of your hand; drink the precious cool liquid; let it refresh you. While you do this, repeat three times:

Affirmation
The great spirit that lives in the water purifies, refreshes, and strengthens my body, mind, and soul.

16

APAN VAYU MUDRA

(Also called the Lifesaver: first aid for heart attacks)

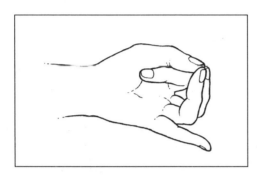

Bend your index finger and let its tip touch the ball of your thumb. At the same time, the tips of the middle and ring fingers touch the tip of your thumb. Extend your little finger. Do this with each hand.

Use as needed until you feel the effect, or practise three times a day for 15 minutes as a course of treatment.

This finger position can have a first-aid function when you use it at the first sign of a heart attack, according to Keshav Dev. It regulates many heart complications. In an emergency, it can even have a quicker effect than placing nitroglycerin (the most frequently used immediate remedy) under the tongue.

Heart attacks, as well as chronic heart complaints, don't just come out of the blue. Instead, they are an indication that a person's lifestyle must be rethought and planned differently. (The Ornish Program has been very successful in this respect.[11]) This mudra can also be used for the general healing and strengthening of the heart.

Heart patients are often so tied up with obligations that they no longer perceive what appears to be "senseless" from the outside. They

---

[11] Dean Ornish, *Dr. Dean Ornish's Program for Reversing Heart Disease* (Random House, 1990).

have no time to relax. They also have a hard time coping with stillness. Something always has to be going on, and they often give so much support to something or someone at work or during their leisure time there is no room for their own needs. Yet, it is precisely these quiet moments that are the ones to nourish our souls. Permit yourself some time for the rosebud image – even if you barely have any to spare. Perhaps you can listen to some music – music that brings you a feeling of lightness – while you do so.

HERBAL REMEDY: Vitamin E in wheatgerm, magnesium, and lemon balm *(Melissa officinalis L.)* also promotes relaxation in the heart.

Imagine a red rosebud in your heart. Whenever you exhale, a petal opens, until the entire flower is completely open. The petals now form a rosette, and the rosette gets a bit larger with every breath until the flower is oversized as it rests upon your chest. You can even feel its weight. Just as your chest rhythmically rises and falls while you breathe, the flower moves as well. Perhaps you can even imagine the fragrance of the rose.

Affirmation
I have the time and the leisure to see beauty and enjoy the silence.

17

BACK MUDRA

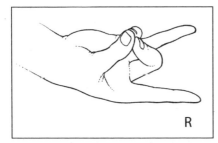

R

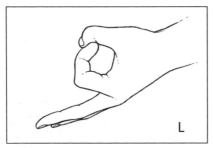

L

Right hand: The thumb, middle finger, and little finger are touching; the index finger and ring finger are extended.

Left hand: Place your thumb joint on the nail of the index finger.

Do four times a day for 4 minutes or, against acute complaints, until it has an effect.

This mudra is primarily effective when someone with a weak back has engaged in an activity (for example: garden work or cleaning) that has strained the back too much and caused painful tensions, or when someone has sat too long in the wrong position. Backaches can have a great variety of causes. Most people have waste deposits and signs of wear, but these don't necessarily have to be painful. A diseased organ whose nerves run through the spinal column can also cause pain. Continuous mental strain, fears, meals that are too heavy, too little sleep, and/or too little exercise are other causes of pain.

This mudra can be even more effective in a position that relieves the back (see illustration on page 93). When doing so, keep the chin pulled in a bit so that the neck is stretched. This little bit of tension has an effect down to the small of the back. After just 20 minutes in this position, the

intervertebral disks are opti-
mally nourished once again
and the metabolism operates
in full swing again. Perhaps
you can even do this exercise
during your lunch break at
the office. Then you can get
through the entire day without pain. What you think

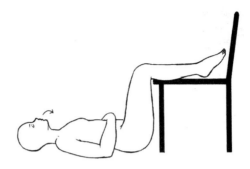

while you do this is also very important, which is why the image and the
affirmation are particularly significant in this position.

HERBAL REMEDY: A massage with St. John's wort oil, olive oil, or
almond oil has a warming and relaxing effect when you suffer from a
backache.

In your mind, you are at a place that does you good – where you feel
well. You are alone, or with people who give you strength and make
you happy. Or you are involved in doing something or engaging in a
sport that you are enthused about. Or you can simply observe your
breathing and pay attention so your thoughts don't drift away.

Affirmation
*My backbone is strong, my back is wide, and I am protected and
supported both inside and outside.*

18

KUBERA MUDRA

(Dedicated to the god of wealth, Kubera)

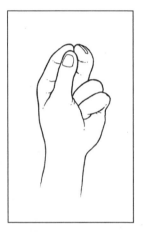

Place the tip of your thumb, index finger, and middle finger together. Bend the other two fingers so they rest in the middle of your hand. Do this with each hand.

The Kubera Mudra can be used for a great variety of concerns. It doesn't matter how long it is practised, but it does matter that you do it with intensity. Many people already know it as the "Three Finger Technique" from Alpha Training[12] and use it when they are looking for something specific – a free parking space, a certain dress, the right book, the necessary information, etc. Others use it when they want to put more force behind their plans for the future. It always involves goals that people want to reach, or wishes that they would like to have fulfilled. With the three closed fingers, additional strength is given to the matter and/or thought. It is obvious that something happens when the fingers of Mars (forcefulness), Jupiter (resplendence, exuberant joy), and Saturn (fixation on the essential and passing through new gateways) join forces. Putting this mudra to specific use in everyday life is quite fun. It also gives us inner repose, confidence, and serenity.

---

[12] Mental Training, which has been developed by Günter and Margarete Friebe. In 1973, this couple studied the methods of Mind Control, Mind Development, and Alphagenics in the USA. During the past twenty years, they have refined these methods so that they now have an independent, very efficient mental training programme.

The practise is simple. In your mind, formulate your wish or goal very clearly into words. Ask your heart whether this is good for you and whether it enriches your surrounding world. Now place the three fingers together, phrase your wish in a positive way as you say it out loud three times. Press your fingers together while you do this. Done! If this concerns a parking spot or a new dress, then the mental preparation isn't as important; otherwise, there are no shortcuts. The following meditation and the affirmation should be done one to two times daily for several days or weeks. This mudra can work wonders, and I'm speaking from my own experience here.

The Kubera Mudra opens and decongests (cleanses) the frontal sinuses, especially if you draw the air upward while inhaling, as if you wanted to smell the fragrance of a flower.

Visualise your goal, your future, or your special wish, in all its colours. At the same time, develop the feeling as if it already were reality. The thought is the procreative power, the father; the feeling is the form-giving power, the mother. Just like large plants need longer to achieve their full bloom, the same applies to our goals and wishes. It is also obvious that we must make our own contribution to this process.

Affirmation
I give my best, and I let the rest be given to me.

19

KUNDALINI MUDRA

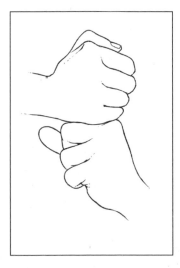

Form a loose fist with both hands. Now extend your left index finger and stick it into the right fist from below. Place the pad of your right thumb on the left finger-tip. Hold the mudra as low as possible in front of your abdomen.

Use as needed or until the desired effect occurs. Or do it three times a day for 15 minutes.

The form of the Kundalini Mudra makes its purpose clear: This is associated with sexual force that is to be awakened or activated. It is the unification of masculine and feminine, the opposites in the polarity. Above all, this mudra symbolises the unification of the individual soul with cosmic soul. The four encircling fingers of the right hand symbolise the outer, perceptible world; the left index finger is our mind and soul, while the thumb represents the Divine.

Sexuality plays a significant role in Tantric Yoga as a spiritual prac-tise. It is important to understand that our sexual organs have a major effect on moods, which is why it's important that these organs be healthy. We should also realise that the desire for sex will change during the course of life. If a person feels no sexual desire, but feels good otherwise, then this is fine and normal. When the desire is there, it should be indulged, either with a partner or alone. This is very important because the secretion that is released in this act has a cleansing function. Bacteria, fungi, etc. that have settled in the vagina are then dissolved and washed out. Many people become ill because they don't yield to their body's natural needs or because they stress themselves by trying to force their bodies to feel desire.

HERBAL REMEDY: Lady's mantle *(Alchemilla xantochlora)* helps as a preventive measure against women's disorders; wild agrimony *(Potentilla anserina L.)* helps against cramplike menstrual complaints.

Just as our sexuality brings us joy and awakens our spirits, as well, the sight of blossoming nature – for pollination can also be seen as a sexual act – imparts new vitality and enthusiasm. Hiking through blossoming meadows, past bubbling streams and fragrant hedges, and through mountain pastures is a nourishing delight for all the senses. Totally luxuriate in these inner pictures. Perhaps we will take the time to enjoy walks in the outside world as well.

Affirmation
I love beauty, and beauty loves me.

20

KSEPANA MUDRA

(The gesture of pouring out and letting go)

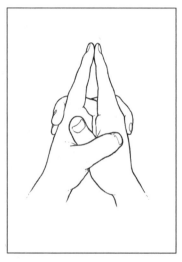

Place your index fingers flat against each other. Clasp the rest of your fingers and let the finger pads rest on the back of your hands. Cross your thumbs and place each in the hollow of the other thumb. There is a small hollow space between your hands. When seated, point the index fingers to the ground. When lying down, point them in the direction of your feet. Completely relax both hands.

Hold this mudra for just 7 to 15 breaths and concentrate on your exhalation. Sigh deeply 3 times while you do this. Then, place your hands on your thighs with palms turned upward.

The Ksepana Mudra stimulates elimination through the large intestine, skin (perspiration), and lungs (improves exhalation), as well as removing expended energies. It should not be held for too long, because fresh energy is also caused to flow out after several breaths. In addition, it promotes the release of all types of tension.

When we find ourselves in the midst of many people, we also absorb much of their negative energy – particularly if our own energy level is too low. This mudra encourages expended or negative energy to flow away, followed by the absorption of fresh and positive energy.

HERBAL REMEDY: Done on occasion, a sweat cure also has a cleansing effect, especially if the flu is threatening to break out. After a warm bath, go to bed and drink 2 to 3 cups of linden-flower infusion or elder tea.

Visualise the following picture. You sit on an elevated stone in a stream, or next to it, and hold this mudra. While you exhale, so much sweat pours from every pore that a rivulet flows out of you into the stream. In conclusion, wash yourself in the cooling water of the stream. Then place your hands on your thighs. Turn to the warming sun and let it dry you. Open yourself once again for the fresh energy that fills you anew when you inhale.

Affirmation
Spent energy in my body, mind, and soul flows away from me, and I thankfully accept all things that refresh me.

21

RUDRA MUDRA

(Ruler of the solar plexus chakra)

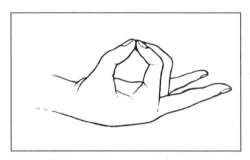

Place the tips of your thumb, index finger, and ring finger together. Extend the other two fingers in a relaxed way. Do this with each hand.

Use as needed, or three to six times a day, for 5 minutes.

Imagine that you are sitting at the centre of a wheel, close to the hub. The wheel can turn as much as it wants, but this has no effect on you. However, when you leave the centre and sit on one of the spokes or at the edge, you must use all of your strength to avoid losing your stability. This applies to all situations in life. When we are not centred, meaning when we are "beside" ourselves, this creates all types of tense states. One individual may have tension in the stomach, another person has tension in the neck, back, pelvis, or chest.

According to the Five Element Theory, the centring force is associated with the earth element (see Appendix C), which rules the energy of the stomach, spleen, and pancreas. The Rudra Mudra strengthens the earth element and its organs. If the chi (the Chinese term for elemental energy) suffers a distinct decrease because of weakened earth energy, there will also be a diminished supply to the head area as a result. Consequently, the person feels listless, heavy, weighed down, or even dizzy. Such a state of weakness can be relieved or even completely eliminated with this mudra.

The Rudra Mudra can also be used by people who have experienced heart complaints, dizziness, the descent of interior organs, or general states of exhaustion.

HERBAL REMEDY: Angelica *(Angelica officinalis Hoffm.)* strengthens the autonomic nervous system and wormwood *(Artemisia absinthium L.)* is the stomach remedy from the herb garden.

The following image will centre your mind by concentrating it on a point, which then increases the power of centring and strengthens body, mind, and soul.

In your mind, see a white canvas in front of you. With a charcoal pencil, draw a wagon wheel on it – the outer rim, the inner rim, and the spokes that connect the inner rim with the outer. The hub is shaped like a square. See a yellow point at the very centre of it. While *inhaling,* let the yellow point come toward you and become increasingly large and shiny. While *exhaling,* let it become smaller again and return to the hub. Always keep your mind focused completely on the centre.

Affirmation
I rest at my centre and draw strength and joy from my centre.

22

GARUDA MUDRA

(Garuda, the mystical bird)

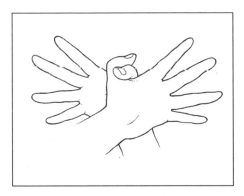

Clasp your thumbs and place your hands, right hand on top of the left hand, on your lower abdomen. Remain in this position for about 10 breaths and then slide your hands up to your navel. Stay there for another 10 breaths. Then place your hands on the pit of your stomach and remain again for about 10 breaths. In conclusion, place your left hand on your sternum, turn your hands in the direction of your shoulders, and spread your fingers.

Do as needed, or three times a day for 4 minutes.

Garuda, the king of birds and of the air, is the enemy of the snakes. This is the powerful and mighty bird that Vishnu rides. Birds generally have sharp eyes, a distinct sense of orientation, and strong survival instincts. Large birds have such an enormous wing span and so much strength in their wings that they can let themselves be carried by the wind.

The Garuda Mudra is very powerful and should be dosed well. This mudra activates blood flow and circulation, invigorates the organs, and balances energy on both sides of the body. Whether in the pelvic or chest area, it invigorates and stimulates. It relaxes and relieves pain related to menstrual complaints, stomach upsets, and respiratory difficulties. It also helps people deal with exhaustion and mood fluctuations. Caution is advised for those who have high blood pressure

HERBAL REMEDY: A wonder remedy for blood flow and circulation is arnica *(Arnica montana)*. Never apply arnica to an open wound; it works wonders on bruises.

Try to imagine living your life as a big bird of prey (and not as a poor little mouse). You sail elegantly and lightly through the air and see the landscape (your life) from a certain distance. You see the mountains (your challenges) for what they are (not too high and not too low), and you also see the best way to overcome them. You have the clear sight of a bird of prey and can differentiate between what is significant and what is unimportant. You don't strive to get more or less than you need, and therefore live in contentment and harmony with your surrounding world.

Affirmation
I am inwardly free. I get what is due to me, and I live in harmony with my world.

23

SUCHI MUDRA

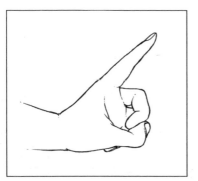

First clench both fists and hold them in front of your chest (basic position). While inhaling, stretch the right arm to the right and point the index finger upward. At the same time, stretch your left arm to the left. Hold this tension for 6 breaths and then return to the basic position. Repeat six times on both sides.

For serious chronic constipation, do four times a day. For light constipation, repeat six to twelve times in the morning and at noon. When traveling or in acute cases, practise every morning before rising for 5 to 10 minutes while comfortably lying in bed. Then hold Mudra Number 24 for several minutes. The Suchi Mudra often helps the first time you do it. If you practise it in the morning at 7, you can usually "unload" before 9.

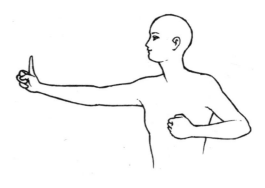

Yogis have always been quite concerned about daily elimination and intestinal cleansing. Unwellness, spite, impatience, violent temper, wanting to cling to everything – the cause for all these unpleasant feelings is often full, and therefore stressed, intestines.

HERBAL REMEDY: Black alder *(Rhamnus frangula)* helps against constipation.

In your mind, see yourself as a generous person, as someone who likes to give unconditionally, and wisely, and who liberally distributes an appropriate portion of your income. See yourself as someone who can also forgive yourself and your fellow human beings; who can toss out old prejudices and other figments of the mind, and risk having new experiences; and who starts every day as a new person with fresh vigour. Let this inner concept become increasingly true in your outer world.

Affirmation
I let go and give up everything that has been used up in my body, mind, and soul.

24

MUSHTI MUDRA

(Fist)

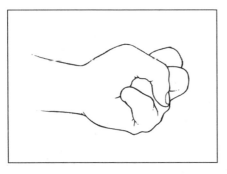

Bend your fingers inward and place your thumbs over the ring fingers. Do this with each hand.

Do as needed, or three times a day for 15 minutes.

The Mushti Mudra activates the liver and stomach energy, promotes digestion, and helps cure constipation.

When we show someone our fist, the other person understands this gesture and will react with fear, flight, or counterattack. But this will hardly solve the problem. Unfortunately, this is why aggression has become so disreputable, and many people suppress it to the extent that they hardly even perceive it around them. Immediately living out every aggression in a wild way certainly isn't good either, but neither is suppressing it. We can reduce aggression to a large extent when we find out its cause. There is blind fury and righteous anger – but there are worlds between them. The cause of many physical complaints, such as a weak liver, problems with digestion or constipation, tension, heart complaints, etc., are related to suppressed or uncontrolled aggression. Most aggression is based on not being able to say "no," not being able to set boundaries, letting oneself be driven into a corner, etc. The basic evil is fear.

When aggression arises, it should be let out in the foreseeable future. Make vigorous fists and punch pillows with them, jog, stomp, dance, or even clean the house! Then look for the cause of the aggression and develop a strategy as to how its trigger can be eliminated. Many problems can be cleared up by discussing them.

HERBAL REMEDY: The herb against stress, which has been scientifically proved, is taiga root *(Eleutherococcus senticosus Maximowicz)*.

Imagine scenes in which you behave too fearfully or too aggressively. Now change the scenes to how you would like them to be. For example, you can practise how to say "no" or how you act toward a boss, your partner, or your parents. But just saying "no" doesn't achieve all that much: mentally work out sensible suggestions for solutions. Whether in planning the weekend or restructuring work, you can train your clear powers of imagination and awaken your fantasy in this respect. Your life will soon be more colourful and richer.

Affirmation
I am quiet and serene in every situation.

25

MATANGI MUDRA

(Matangi – god of inner harmony and royal rulership)

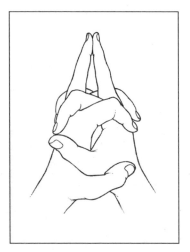

Fold your hands in front of your solar plexus (stomach area), point both middle fingers and place against each other. Direct your attention to the breath in the solar plexus or stomach area.

Do as needed, or three times a day for 4 minutes.

This mudra strengthens the breathing impulse in the solar plexus and balances the energies in this area. It stimulates the wood element, which represents new beginnings, and the earth element, which gives life its depth. The heart, stomach, liver, duodenum, gallbladder, spleen, pancreas, and kidneys profit from the Matangi Mudra. An excited heart becomes noticeably more calm, and inner tension (such as diverse spasms or sensations of fullness) that hamper digestion are resolved. According to Kim da Silva, this mudra also relieves vague pain and tension in the jaw.

HERBAL REMEDY: Lavender *(Lavandula angustifolia Miller)* and verbena *(Verbena officinalis)* are herbs of repose and harmony.

Green and yellow are the colours of the solar plexus. Yellow lightens our mood and stimulates the mind. Green is the colour of harmony. Each of us needs an inner place (a retreat) where we can go to be safe. We can create this place inside ourselves. If we can get there without using any physical means of transportation, we also don't pollute our environment and can really save time.

Imagine a yellow desert in which you create a beautiful green oasis, a place of harmony and joy. This is your personal retreat, and you form it completely according to your own preferences and needs. Here you find yourself again. You become calm and still, and your soul attains peace.

Affirmation
Rest, silence, and peace fill me completely.

26

MAHASIRS MUDRA

(Large head mudra)

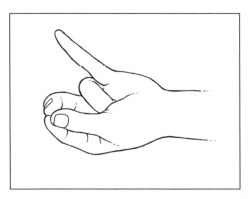

The tips of your thumb, index finger, and middle finger touch each other. Place your ring finger into the fold of the thumb and keep your little finger extended. Do this with each hand.

Do as needed, or three times every day for 6 minutes.

Headaches have a great variety of causes and can hardly be made to disappear once and for all with one single mudra. Frequently, weather influences or tension in the eyes, neck, back, or pelvis are at fault; or there are problems with the sinuses or digestion. All of this can result in too much energy being focused on the head, and this leads to tension that causes pain in the head. In order to release this tension, it is important to direct consciousness into other body parts (abdomen, feet, or hands). The Mahasirs Mudra balances energy, has a tension-relieving effect, and eliminates mucous congestion in the frontal sinuses.

If you have the time to lie down, try out these additional measures against headaches. Dip a washcloth in water that has some vinegar added to it, lie down, and place the washcloth on your feet. The soles, the backs of the feet, and the toes should be packed well. Now massage up and down your neck by vigorously pressing your index and middle fingers into the middle of the nape of your neck, then massage both frontal eminences (bumps on both sides of the forehead), and finally form the Mahasirs Mudra with your fingers.

HERBAL REMEDY: You can drink a tea made from willow bark *(Salix alba),* meadowsweet *(Filipendula ulmaria),* or feverfew *(Chrysanthemum parthenium).* In order to prevent a migraine, you can do an enema.

While exhaling, imagine that waves of energy are flowing down from your head through your neck, back, arms, and legs, and leaving through your hands and feet. After a while, imagine that your head is clear, cool, clean, and light. In conclusion, stroke your face with spread fingers and enjoy the feeling for a while.

Affirmation
I have a free, light, clear, and cool head.

27

HAKINI MUDRA

(Hakini – god of the Forehead [6th] Chakra)

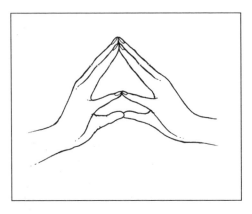

Place all the fingertips together.

The Hakini Mudra can be practised at any time.

When you would like to remember something, or want to find the red thread again, place your fingertips together, direct your eyes upward, place the tip of your tongue on your gums while inhaling, and let the tongue fall again while exhaling. Then take a deep breath – and what you wanted should immediately occur to you. Moreover, when you must concentrate on something for a longer period of time, could use some good ideas, or want to remember something that you have read, this mudra can be useful. When doing mental work, don't cross your feet. Sit with your eyes facing west. This mudra can do true wonders, and you should always keep it in the back of your mind in case of an emergency.

In terms of science, this finger position has been researched quite well; researchers have determined that it promotes the cooperation between the right and left brain hemispheres. It is also recommended today in memory training and management courses. It is said to open access to the right hemisphere, which is where the memory is stored. This mudra also improves and deepens respiration, and the brain profits from it as well. In order to recharge the brain's energy, you can practise the Maha

Bandha (see page 171) or use these fragrance essences – lemon, rosemary, basil, or hyssop.

According to Kim da Silva, the Hakini Mudra builds up the energy of the lungs. To activate the energy of the large intestine, shift the finger contact by one finger so that the right index finger is on the left thumb, your right middle finger is on your left index finger, etc.

HERBAL REMEDY: Lungwort *(Pulmonaria officinalis L.)* benefits the lungs.

You may also improve concentration and gather new mental powers by letting your gaze and thoughts rest on one object or a relaxing activity for a longer period of time. The following exercise also helps in this direction.

About three feet in front of you, imagine an object, such as a burning candle, a piece of fruit, or a stone. Look at the object as long as possible without blinking. Now close your eyes and try to imagine the object. Immediately let go of every rising thought not related directly to the object. Hold your concentration as long as you can.

Affirmation
Concentration is my strength.

28

TSE MUDRA

(Exercise of the three secrets)

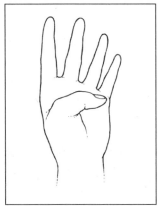

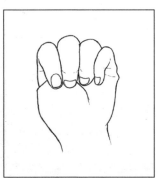

Place both hands on your thighs. Put the thumb tip onto the root of your little finger. Slowly encircle your thumbs with the other four fingers while slowly inhaling through your nose. Hold your breath and form the sound of OM seven times in your head while hearing the vibration of the tone in your right ear.[13] Then slowly exhale while drawing in the abdominal wall; open your hands again and imagine all your worries, fears, and unhappiness leaving your body.

Repeat this exercise seven to forty-nine times, but at least seven times – according to the Taoist monks.

Kim Tawm, an authority on Chinese medicine, writes: "Tradition says that this mudra chases away sadness, reduces fearfulness, turns away misfortune and bad luck, and overcomes depressions. It is known to increase personal magnetism and enhance the intuitive and mental powers."[14]

This is exactly the hand position (thumb in the fist) that I automatically assumed many years ago when I went through my darkest hours, hid-

---

[13] Kim Tawm: *Geheime Übungen taoistischer Mönsche* (Freiburg, 1982), p. 89.
[14] Kim Tawm: *Geheime Übungen taoistischer*, p. 89.

ing on my sofa, weary of life, and very sad. Today it is clear to me that many depressions are caused by the weakness of the water element (see Appendix C), or of the kidney and bladder. This element can actually be restored or recharged like a battery through specific breathing exercises such as those described above.

People who are depressed are frequently given the following advice by the friendly people around them: you should take a walk in the fresh air, do gymnastics, do yoga exercises, etc. However, depressed people often lack the strength to do these things. (I understand this since I know what it means to be in this state.) But since we must always breathe wherever we are, even in the deepest depression, we can at least intensify our breathing (see page 13) and practise the Tse Mudra. Then stretch vigorously. This works wonders!

HERBAL REMEDY: A further wonder remedy against depression is just plain water. Drink a great deal of water and shower frequently. St. John's wort *(Hypericum perforatum L.)* and borage *(Borago officinalis)* are the herbs used to treat depression.

In your mind, see yourself sitting close to the sea. Your feet are gently bathed by the waves. Deeply inhale the refreshing ocean air, hold your breath for a few seconds, and then slowly exhale. Now feel a light rain and how the warm water washes away all your sadness and cares. Then turn your face to the sun and allow the light and warmth to stream in through the pores of your skin. Let yourself be comforted and given new confidence and joy.

Affirmation
I am filled with light, lightness, and divine joy.

29

VAJRA MUDRA

(Gesture of the fiery thunderbolt)

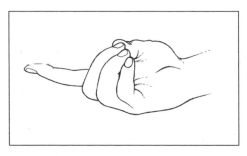

Press your thumb onto the side of the middle fingernail, the ring finger on the other side of your middle fingernail, and the little finger at the side of your ring fingernail. Extend your index finger. Do this with each hand.

Do as needed, or three times a day for 5 minutes.

In addition, relief can be obtained by massaging the root of the nose, the centre of the forehead, the back of the head, and the nape of the neck with the middle finger.

Circulation may be weakened when blood pressure is too low, or there is a weakness in the earth element (see Appendix C), which is associated with the energy of the stomach, spleen, and pancreas, or a weak heart. A lack of drive, listlessness, and dizziness are the consequences.

With the Vajra Mudra, you can stimulate circulation. The back bends and side bends of yoga (see pages 182 and 186) also activate these respective energies. Walking at a brisk pace, listening to lively or exciting music (such as Beethoven's *Hammerklavier* Piano Sonata and the 1st, 2nd, 5th, or 7th Symphony; George Gerschwin's Piano Concert in F Major; jazz or rock 'n' roll, march music, techno, etc.) can also give you new drive. In addition, pouring very warm or cold water onto your wrists can also help. *Caution:* A lack of drive can come from extreme physical or mental-emotional fatigue: rest and recuperation are then necessary. Do not use any type of stimulant in this case!

HERBAL REMEDY: Nature's major stimulants are arnica *(Arnica montana)* and rosemary *(Rosmarinus officinalis)*.

Imagine a fiery, glowing ball in your pelvis. With every inhalation, the fireball climbs up your spinal column, to your heart, through the throat, and up into your skull. The ball heats your body and your vitality; it warms your heart and illuminates your mind.

Affirmation
I enjoy this present day with joy in my heart.

BHRAMARA MUDRA

(The bee)

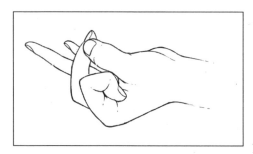

Place your index finger in the thumb fold, and the tip of your thumb on the side of your middle fingernail. Extend your ring and little fingers. Do this with each hand.

Do four times a day for 7 minutes. If you have more time, you can hold the Bhramara Mudra up to eight times a day for about 20 minutes. The name of this mudra comes from Indian dance and represents the bee. Today we use bee products against allergies, and this mudra has the same effect.

The cause of allergies is a weakened immune system and/or intestinal flora that has also been affected. For example, antibiotics and many other medications harm the intestinal flora. The effects are mucous congestion in the frontal sinuses, bronchial tubes, and intestinal tract, not to mention a great variety of rashes. A change of weather, pollen, and animal hairs are often just the triggers, but not the actual cause. I used to experience a routine alternation between asthma and allergies. Today I live without the symptoms of these disorders because I have changed my diet and lifestyle. It is best for people who have allergies to eat little or no (even better!) meat, tomatoes, hot peppers, kiwis, and strawberries, and they should not drink milk.

To strengthen the immune system, a routine programme of yoga, jogging, or hiking is helpful. Reducing stress and getting enough rest is also important. Treating it with healing earth can restore the healthy intestinal flora.

Enemas are very effective, and not as complicated as they may seem. Hang a water container (or special enema bag available from the pharmacy) above the bathtub, fill it with lukewarm sage or chamomile tea, kneel down in the bathtub in the cat posture (see page 80), and gently guide the (lubricated) end of the hose into the anus. Then let all the tea water run into the large intestine. The rest will take care of itself. Repeat three times and then rest for a while. It is best to do the enema every other day during one week. That should suffice for several months at a time.

People with allergies often have a cleanliness mania, or they are afraid of contagious diseases. Become aware of your fears and work on dissolving them by taking a mental look at what triggers fear.

What are you afraid of? Imagine an object to which you are allergic. And then imagine how to stay healthy when you touch it. At first, you may feel inner resistance against this idea, which is normal. Repeat the images until you react neutrally to them.

Affirmation
In love and serenity, I like [name].

31

UTTARABODHI MUDRA

(Mudra of the highest enlightenment)

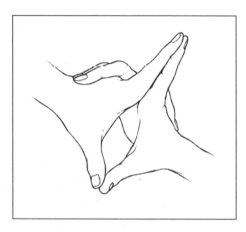

Place both hands folded in front of your solar plexus, at the level of your stomach. Lay the respective index fingers and thumbs on each other. Point your index fingers upward to the ceiling, and your thumbs downward to the floor or stomach. If you are lying down, the tips of your thumbs may lie at the lower end of your sternum.

The Uttarabodhi Mudra can be held anywhere, at any time, and for as long as you want.

You can use this mudra when you feel physically and mentally listless, when you want to relax, or when you need a rousing idea – a flash of inspiration.

The Uttarabodhi Mudra strengthens the metal element (see Appendix C), which is associated with the energy of the lungs and large intestine. It strengthens inhalation; and since the heart and upper lung areas are particularly opened when this mudra is done, it has a refreshing effect. The metal element has a direct relationship with the nervous system and anything that conducts electrical and/or energetic impulses. These are both the internal and external paths that connect human beings with the surrounding world and the cosmic forces. The metal element conducts the universal life force, also called *chi* or *prana,* from the outside to the inside and is also responsible for charging the inner power reservoirs. I like to compare this mudra with a lightning rod, and I practise it frequently before I give a talk, teach a class, or write. On the one hand, I want to make a connection with the divine powers that should be the essence of my work; and on the other hand, I would like to create the connection for the listeners, students, and/or readers. Test the effect of this mudra – you will be amazed!

HERBAL REMEDY: Sallow thorn *(Hippophae rhamnoides L.)*, which is to be taken during the dark winter months in particular, refreshes body, mind, and soul.

Imagine a line that extends from your pelvis to your heart, your head, and far beyond your head, losing itself in infinity. Whatever you now desire – solutions, answers, healing power, clarity, etc. – comes to you through this line as light from the cosmos. Perhaps you also wish for something for a fellow human being. Then conduct this light into your heart and to the respective person from there.

Affirmation
*My partnership with the powers of the cosmos allows my life
to appear in a new light.*

32

DETOXIFICATION MUDRA

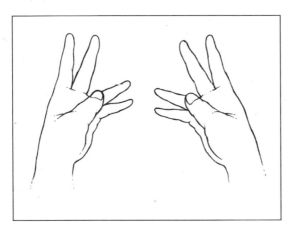

Place each thumb on the inner edge of the third joint of your ring finger. Do this with each hand. At least once a year, we should all plan a detoxification treatment. It makes no difference whether this is done at a beautiful spa or at home. The important thing is to pamper yourself, and allow yourself rest during this time, while still getting some exercise (walking, yoga, breathing exercises). A rice or potato treatment has a very efficient but gentle effect. For three to five days, eat easily digestible bread with herb tea made of stinging nettle *(Urtica dioica L.)* in the morning; for lunch and dinner, have a meal of rice or potatoes and steamed leaf vegetables. Drink tea or water between meals. Do an enema (see page 119) every second day and occasionally support the detoxification process with a compress. For example, a potato compress is quite easy to use and practically draws the toxins out of the body. It can be used to support general cleansing by placing it on the liver or any other body parts that hurt. Boil the potatoes in their skins and mash with a fork, wrap in a cotton towel, and place on the body; wrap a warm towel around the body and the potato sack. Leave the compress on the respective spot for about 30 minutes.

During the detoxification days, lie down to rest often. This is the time to use this mudra for supporting the detoxification process. It is important to consider the things, in addition to waste materials and toxins, you are willing to let go of – bad memories, old grudges, bad habits, negative character traits, fears, etc. This will make room for something new. What should it be?

Do the following visualisation several times a day, with enthusiasm!

Visualise a film where you see what you are letting go of. Allow yourself enough time to do this. Afterward, visualise new qualities that you desire. Imagine everything new in a very lively and detailed manner; create within yourself the feelings (relief, pride, joy, etc.) that you will have when the goal has been reached – when your wish is fulfiled.

Affirmation
I entrust my wish or goal to divine protection – and everything will be fine.

33

SHAKTI MUDRA

(In honour of Shakti, the goddess of life energy)

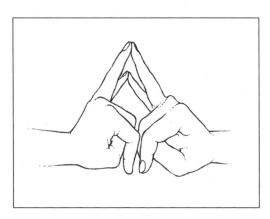

Place your ring fingers and little fingers together. The other fingers are loosely bent over your thumbs, which are placed in your palm. Focus on your breathing in the pelvic area, and slow down exhalation somewhat.

Do as needed, or three times a day for 12 minutes.

The Shakti Mudra intensifies the respiratory impulse in the lower chest area. You can increasingly perceive breathing in the pelvic area. It has a calming effect and will help you fall asleep at night. If it is done too often or held for too long, it may also lead to lethargy. It can bring pleasant relaxation to the pelvic area. As a result, it can counteract spasms in the intestines, or even menstrual complaints.

I am frequently asked for advice about difficulties in falling asleep. One of the following tips always works:

- Practise this mudra in a slightly different form before trying to sleep. If you sleep on your sides, you can take a corner of the pillow between your hands, place the little fingers and ring fingers together, and let the others lay on or beneath the pillow.

- Bend one hand back and slowly turn it to the left and to the right six times; then do the other hand; then one foot, and then the other.
- Moisten the outer and inner sides of your legs with a wet cloth; go to bed without drying them.

HERBAL REMEDY: Valerian *(Valeriana officinalis L.)* and hops *(Humulus lupulus L.)* also have a calming effect.

Colour combinations in green and soft, flowing forms always have a calming effect. Visualise green pictures (a landscape, leaves, a silk scarf, etc.) and let your exhalation become increasingly slower and deeper while you do so.

Affirmation
Silence, harmony, and peace fill my entire being.

34

MAHA SACRAL MUDRA

(Large pelvis mudra)

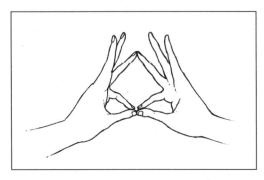

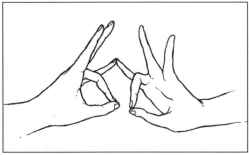

Place your ring finger pads together, with your little fingers on the thumbs. Hold this hand position for 10 breaths.

Now place the pads of your little fingers together, and place your ring fingers on your thumbs. Also hold this variation for 10 breaths.

Do as needed, or three times a day for 7 minutes.

This wonderful mudra helps handle complaints in the lower abdomen; it is particularly good against pain during menstruation. It can also bring relief for inactive intestines, intestinal spasms, or bladder and prostate complaints, since it has a relaxing and energy-balancing effect.

While holding this mudra, you can additionally practise the Maha Bandha (see page 172) ten to thirty times. Repeat several times each day. This exercise can naturally also be practised while sitting on the toilet.

The secret afflictions of many people are bladder weakness, hemorrhoids, and atony or tension in the area of the bladder and anus. These problems can be relieved by training the PC muscle.[15] As an additional measure against weakness of the bladder and anal sphincter, Viparita Karani (see page 188) can be used.

HERBAL REMEDY: Chewing pumpkin seeds and drinking pear *(Pyrus communis)* or bearberry leaf *(Arctostaphylos uva-ursi)* tea are also good for the bladder.

Problems with elimination are often also accompanied by mental and emotional difficulties about letting go in general, or with fear of having to go through something. You can build up positive patterns in this respect with the following image.

Doesn't the world always look a bit friendlier on the other side of a long tunnel? We frequently have to pass through tunnels in life – we have to go through something. The image of a tunnel that we walk through can help us keep going, carry on, and be hopeful. Every tunnel ultimately takes us to the light, but we need the courage and strength to go through it to the end.

Affirmation
No matter how dark my path may be at times, it leads to light.

---

[15] Puboccygenus muscle in the perineum between the anus and the genital organs. After extensive studies, researchers have come to the conclusion that tensing this muscle has the effect of an energy pump on the brain.

35

MAKARA MUDRA

(Makara – the name of a crocodile in Indian mythology)

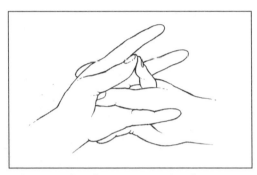

Place one hand inside the other. Extend the thumb of your lower hand through the little finger and ring finger of the other and place in the middle of the palm of your upper hand. This hand's thumb and the tip of your ring finger touch each other. Do this three times a day for 4 to 10 minutes.

Within the shortest amount of time, the crocodile can mobilse tremendous strength, which it has built up during its endlessly long resting periods. Human beings also have reserves of strength that are restored during phases of rest. This mudra activates kidney energy, which is related to this reserve of strength. Feeling listless, depressed, and dissatisfied – as well as having black rings under your eyes – usually indicates a reduced supply of energy. In addition to walking in the fresh air, and getting ear massages, the breathing exercises of yoga are also helpful here. I have found the complete yoga breath – which can be practised while standing, walking, sitting, or lying down – to be quite effective. To do this, breathe in deeply, arch your abdominal and chest area forward, draw up your shoulders. Hold your breath for several seconds and then slowly exhale. At the end of the exhalation, pull in the abdominal wall a bit so that even more air is squeezed out. When doing this, *be sure to hold the pauses after inhalation and exhalation for several seconds.* Despite this, keep the breath slow, regular, and fine. This mudra has a calming and centring effect, giving you a sense of security and confidence.

HERBAL REMEDY: The birch *(Betula verrucosa)*, which sucks up to 70 quarts of water from the ground every day and evaporates it through the leaves, helps against renal function impairment. Goldenrod *(Solidago virgaurea L.)* is effective against pyelitis, and ground ivy *(Glechoma hederacea L.)* eases nervous bladder complaints.

The colour blue has a positive influence on the water element.

Visualise a meadow filled with blue flowers. Behind it, you see the blue ocean with a blue sky arched above it.

Affirmation
Cosmic, divine energy is completely available to me at any time and place, and I use it wisely.

36

MUKULA MUDRA

(Beak hand)

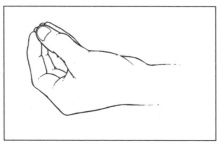

Place the four fingers on your thumbs and put your fingertips on the part of your body that needs more energy. Do this with each hand.

Do as needed, or five times a day for 5 minutes.

This energy-giving and relaxing mudra is placed on the organ or body part that hurts, or that feels weak or tense. This is like directing a laser ray of regenerating energy to the respective body part or organ that needs healing. Samuel West, an American scientist and healer, uses the Mukula Mudra when he wants to electrically recharge an organ, and has been very successful with this method. He was able to prove that every health disorder, as well as many undefinable pains, is caused because the respective electrical field is too weak. According to West, the fingers should be placed on the various organs as follows:

Lungs: Place your fingers on the right side and left side, about 2 inches below the collarbone.

Stomach: Place the fingers of both hands directly beneath the sternum.

Liver and gallbladder: Place your left hand at the lower end of the sternum. With your right hand, stroke 21 times across the ends of the ribs on the right side, as if you wanted to light a match.

Spleen and pancreas: Place your right hand at the lower end of the sternum. With your left hand, stroke 21 times across the ends of the ribs on the left side, as if you wanted to light a match.

Kidneys: Place the fingers of both hands about two inches above the waist on the back.

Bladder: Place the fingers of both hands on the right and left side of the abdomen, next to the pubic bone.

Intestines: Place the fingers of one hand on the navel and, from right to left, draw a circle that becomes increasingly larger (like a spiral).[16]

Always do a complete yoga breath while you do this. After inhaling, during the extended pause, say the affirmation below.

The following colours achieve an additional effect:

For treatment of the lungs, visualise the colour white; for the liver and gallbladder, green; for the stomach, spleen, and pancreas, use yellow; use red for the heart or small intestine; use blue for the kidneys and bladder.

Affirmation
Dirt out – power in.

---

[16] Jo Conrad and Benjamin Seiler, "Atmen Sie sich gesund" in *ZeitenSchrift* 5/95, p. 5.

37

JOINT MUDRA

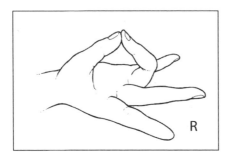

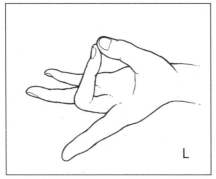

Right hand: Thumb and ring finger together.

Left hand: Thumb and middle finger together.

Do as needed, or four times a day for 15 minutes. In case of illness, the mudra should be held six times a day for 30 minutes.

This mudra balances energy in your joints. I have had very good experience with it when my knees were sore after a hike, especially walking down mountains, or when I have worked too long at the computer and have an unpleasant feeling in my elbows.

There are many dynamic yoga exercises you can use to help against joint pain. These can be found in my *Basic Yoga for Everybody* (a book and card set published by Weiser in 1999). All of the older relatives in my family are afflicted to some extent by severe arthrosis. Twenty years ago, I also suffered from pain in the knee and hip joints. Today, thanks to yoga, I have no more symptoms. All types of compresses are also helpful – just don't let anyone talk you into believing that the situation is chronic and you now have to suffer from such pain for the rest of your life. Do something to counteract it! The healing may take months, but if you are persistent, you can have success with it.

A wonderful exercise for all the joints is the Little Bear (see illustration). It is important to do the circles very loosely and slowly. Slow down the flow of your breath when you do the movements.

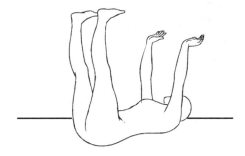

Lie on your back, draw your chin in slightly, and hug your knees. Then move the legs and arms into a vertical position.

- Shake both hands and feet to relax them.
- Circle your foot and hand joints.
- Draw wide circles with your arms and legs, as if you wanted to draw a big infinity sign on the ceiling.
- Bend and stretch your legs and arms.

HERBAL REMEDY: The herb for joints, whether human or animal, has always been comfrey *(Symphytum officinale L.)*.

Visualise images where you completely enjoy your flexibility; you easily and freely move your legs and arms, feet and hands, head and neck. You see yourself as a dancer, athlete, or performer and feel how your energy flows and your mood improves.

Affirmation
I enjoy my flexibility. It uplifts my soul and stimulates my mind.

38

KALESVARA MUDRA

(Dedicated to the deity Kalesvara, who rules over time)

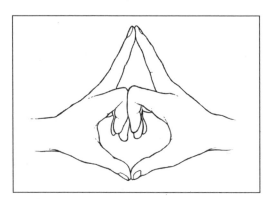

Place the finger pads of your middle finger together; touch the first two joints of the index fingers and touch your thumbs. Bend your other fingers inward. Point your thumbs toward your chest and spread your elbows to the outside.

Inhale and exhale slowly 10 times. Then observe your breath and lengthen the pause after inhalation and after exhalation a little bit more.

The Kalesvara Mudra calms the flood of thoughts; it calms agitated feelings. The more calm we become, the longer the time periods between the thoughts. We become more clear; we make new observations about ourselves; we can seek and find solutions.

This mudra can also be used to help change character traits, support memory and concentration, or eliminate addictive behaviour. It should be practised at least 10 to 20 minutes a day for these purposes.

As long as we live, we work on our character traits, much like a stonecutter hews a sculpture out of a lump of stone. This shouldn't be a battle, but loving and understanding guidance that pushes us in the right direction. As unpleasant and uncomfortable as bad character traits, habits, or addictions may be, they also help us progress when we overcome them.

HERBAL REMEDY: When the mind is overly active, when certain thoughts circle in the mind and cannot be put aside, I find Bach Flower No. 35 (White Chestnut) to work true wonders.

- First ask about the benefit that this characteristic or habit brings.
- Ask the cosmic consciousness for help and partnership in this project.
- Describe the new characteristic or habit as precisely as possible.

Now imagine scenes in which you act and react in a new way.

Affirmation
I enjoy being [like this and like that].

39

SHIVALINGA

(Energy-charging Mudra)

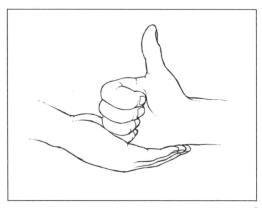

Place your right hand, with thumb extended upward, on top of your left hand, which is shaped like a bowl. Hold the fingers of your left hand close together. Position your hands at the level of the abdomen, with your elbows pointing outward and slightly forward.

Do as often as you like, or two times a day for 4 minutes.

The right hand in this mudra symbolises the masculine force – Shiva's phallus. Shiva embodies the destructive and transformative aspect of the highest deity in Indian mythology. Just as the phallus is the symbol of a new beginning, Shiva is the deity who makes this new beginning possible in the first place by destroying something, thereby creating the necessary preconditions. If, for example, flowers wouldn't wilt, there would also be no fruit. Or, if the spent cells within us were not destroyed, there would be proliferations. It is an eternal cycle and must function perfectly within us on the physical and mental-emotional levels. An inner force keeps it going, and each of us has this force within our reservoir, which is associated with the water element (see Appendix C). The breath nourishes this reservoir of energy. This is why the optimal quality of the breath (see page 13) is so important. The water element has its effect on the outer edge of the hand and the palm, and the thumb is like an inflow for energy, which is absorbed through the lungs.

This mudra can be used against tiredness, dissatisfaction, listlessness, and depression. Or we can use it when we feel drained because of long periods of tension or strain. You can do it while you are waiting, such as while waiting for the doctor's findings. This mudra helps the healing process, no matter where we are sick. In terms of healing, this mudra is responsible for many more wonders than people know. Keep this fact in the back of your mind when you need healing.

Imagine that your left hand is a mortar and your right hand is a pestle. During the first breaths, mentally let whatever makes you sick fall like dark pebbles into your left hand. With the edge of your right hand, grind everything into the finest dust, which you then blow away from your hand like fine sand. Afterward, remain seated for a while and let healing energy flow into the bowl formed by your hand (your energy reservoir) through the right thumb. Fervently speak the following affirmation several times.

Affirmation
Healing light illuminates every cell of my body, dissolves everything that should be dissolved, and builds up what must be built up again.
Thank you!

40

DYNAMIC MUDRA

As the name already implies, during this mudra the fingers are not held still, but are moved.

During each *exhalation,* place one of your fingertips on the tip of your thumb; while *inhaling,* extend the fingers again. Speak a syllable mantra while doing this (see example below). Do this with each hand. (You can start on the exhale as you can only inhale when you have exhaled.)

During "saaa," press together the thumb and index finger;
During "taaa," use middle finger and thumb;
During "naaa," use ring finger and thumb;
During "maaa," use little finger and thumb.

When you do it the *second* time, press your fingernail instead of your fingertip with your thumb.

During the *third* time, press your whole finger with the thumb. At the same time, press your fingertip into the palm of the hand.

This mudra can be practised every day for 5 to 30 minutes.

When we were children, we played finger games in which the individual fingers were pressed, bent, or extended according to the lines of a nursery rhyme. Today, physical therapists and educators use these hand exercises for speech and/or learning difficulties. This is a wonderful mudra for promoting brain activity and relaxing the nerves. It promotes concentration and creates inner relaxation. Please be sure that you breathe slowly, that you inhale and exhale evenly and in a relaxed way.

41

JNANA MUDRA AND CHIN MUDRA

(Gesture of consciousness and gesture of knowledge)

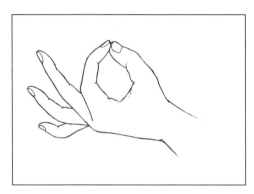

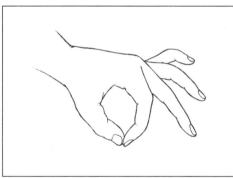

Place the tip of the thumb on your index fingertip and extend your other fingers. Lay your hand on your thigh in a relaxed way. Do this with each hand.

When your fingers point up to Heaven, it is called the *Jnana Mudra;* when your fingers point down to Earth, it is called the *Chin Mudra.*

The mudra is done in two different ways. The first way, as described above, allows the tips of your thumb and index finger to touch each other; for the second variation, the tip of your index finger touches the first thumb joint (shown in the illustration on page 140), and the thumb places light pressure on the nail of your index finger. The first variation is the passive receiving position; the second one is an actively giving position.

These are the two best-known hand positions of Hatha Yoga, and they have an effect on the physical, mental, emotional, and spiritual level.

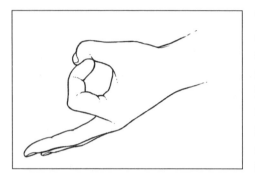

These gestures symbolise the connected nature of human consciousness (thumbs). The three extended fingers symbolise the three *gunas* – traits that keep evolution in both microcosm and macrocosm in motion: *tamas* (lethargy), *rajas* (activity), and *sattwa* (balance and harmony). The closed circle of the index finger and thumb depict the actual goal of yoga – the unification of *Atman,* the individual soul, with *Brahman*, the world soul.

We find this mudra in many of the Hindu portrayals of deities; in them, the right hand is raised to the heart, and the thumb and index finger, which touch each other, are facing the believer. It is the gesture of proclaiming a teaching. The Buddhists are also familiar with the gesture and call it the *Vitarka Mudra* (discussion gesture). With this gesture, the deity or Buddha underline the meaning of the words. Christ was also depicted on old Byzantine icons using this gesture; in Catholic liturgy, the priest makes the same gesture after the transubstantiation.

I also find it beautiful when the Jnana Mudra is practiced at the heart. Raise your hand to the level of the heart, letting the index finger and thumb touch. Here they should be directed inward and upward. Here they simply symbolise the wisdom of God. This is the devotion of the human being to divine wisdom and its recognition. There is also a certain tenderness in this gesture that touches my heart.

With these variations of the Jnana Mudra, we already find ourselves on the spiritual level. However, the physical effect should not be overlooked. When this gesture is employed to heal physical complaints, it makes no difference whether the Jnana Mudra or the Chin Mudra is practised. According to Keshav Dev, this mudra is a universal remedy for improving states of mental tension and disorder, as well as for promoting memory and concentration. It clears the mind – and we all want to have a "clear head" in any situation. It is also used for insomnia, as well as sleepiness, depression, and high blood pressure. This mudra can be combined with other mudras and enhances their effects when practised before or after them. You can hold the gesture with just your right hand, and practise another mudra with your left hand. You will find further uses for this mudra on page 6.

This mudra activates the metal element (see Appendix C) and is associated with the colour white. White is the apparent void in which fullness is concealed. White is the colour of birth and death, of a new beginning and completion. White is also the colour of unity and peace. White clears the mind and brings peace to the soul.

Visualise the colour white. First do this by mentally looking at a white object, then do it abstractly. Visualise a white wall and let yourself be surprised by the forms and colours that descend upon you. There may be encoded messages hidden in them.

Affirmation
Divine knowledge makes my life richer and easier; divine wisdom gladdens my heart and shows me the path.

SPIRITUAL MUDRAS

*T*he following mudras have been used in temples and churches since time immemorial to support meditation or prayer. They can always be seen in the Hindu depictions of the gods, as well as in portrayals of Christ, Buddha, and the saints. The hand position of the respective deities or sages expresses an inner state of mind as well; the meditating person hopes, either consciously or unconsciously, to also enter into the appropriate mood. The mudras symbolise characteristics that we hope to acquire. After long meditative observation, people can take on these characteristics. Another example of this principle is that after looking at the many sculptures of the gods, visitors to museums in Greece assume a more upright posture themselves.

I believe that spirituality should be integrated into everyday life, plans for the future, and coming to terms with the past. Consequently, I have also included in this chapter newer mudras that address the habits of thought and feeling.

There is usually no indication of how long the mudras should be done here since this is different for each individual. One person may need to do the following mudra meditations just once, and for only a few minutes to feel their effects – depending on the level of inner maturity; other people may have to meditate for several days or even weeks, from 7 to 30 minutes a day, before they even perceive that something has changed or that their connection with higher consciousness has deepened.

42

ATMANJALI MUDRA

(Gesture of prayer)

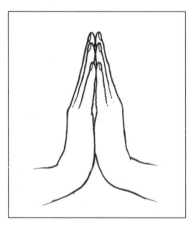

Place both hands together in front of your heart chakra. Leave a little hollow space between the two palms. At the beginning or close of the meditation, sit or stand for a while with your arms spread and raised to Heaven.

Placing your hands together in front of your chest supports inner collection and creates harmony, balance, repose, silence, and peace. This gesture activates and harmonises coordination of the left and right brain hemispheres. It can support a supplicatory meditation when you have a request of the Divine, when you have a heart's desire that you would like to have fulfilled. With this gesture, you also express reverence or gratitude. In India, it is a gesture of greeting or thanks; it shows respect for fellow human beings.

The ancient Celts and Teutons contacted their gods with raised arms. This gesture is very powerful and was prohibited during Christianisation. Later, it was introduced once again. However, only the priests and members of religious orders – but no longer the common people – were permitted to use it. Who was meant to have the power here? In India and Nepal, people make this gesture toward holy people and to those they respect.

As already mentioned, this mudra calms our thoughts and creates clarity as a result. Calming thoughts are always based on a certain power, a power that builds up physical strength and stabilises the mind, as well as clarifying and strengthening.

Imagine that you are at a holy place of power. Perhaps you know of a holy place of power that has special meaning for you. Then, in your thoughts, you can bring it to the privacy of your own room at any time. You can also visualise a place that harmonises with your needs. Imagine this place as precisely as possible. At holy places, we feel a special energy. Try to also feel this energy within yourself. This mudra will bring you to the silence; whether you make a request, ask a question, give praise, or give thanks – if you are willing to be helped, you are certain to be helped at the right time and in the best way possible. At the end of the meditation, remain in silence for a while. Immerse yourself in the peace and joy of the Divine.

Affirmation
Full of thankfulness, I receive the good that waits for me.

43

DHYANI MUDRA

(Gesture of meditation – of contemplation)

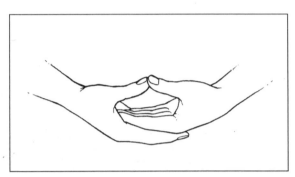

Place both hands like bowls in your lap. The left hand lies in the right hand and the thumbs touch each other.

This is the classical meditation pose, and I assume it whenever I meditate without any special intentions. When I simply sit and observe my breath, I am completely passive and let the divine force act within me and for me. I know that the Divine wants only the best for me and helps me at any time and place if I allow it. "Your will be done," is an expression of most heartfelt joy.

The two hands formed into a bowl show that we are inwardly free, pure, and empty in order to receive everything that we need on our spiritual path. Since there is no empty space in the universe (everything that appears "empty" to us is full of subtle energy), this void will become filled with new energy – our thoughts and feelings determine the quality. This is why it is so important to have done the work of forgiveness beforehand and live in peace with all beings.

It is also like a silent cooperation with your best friend. You no longer need to tell each other anything – you are content because you know that everything important has already been said. You feel the connection, and that is enough.

In classical meditation, emptiness is brought to mind with this mudra, meaning you think of nothing at all. This is very difficult; consequently, there is also a second version. Here the attention is directed at breathing – all the senses are focused on the breath. This is more likely to work, yet there may still be difficulties with it. If your thoughts stray too often from your breathing, or if you feel the smallest tendency toward negative brooding . . .

. . . then imagine a symbol for the Divine (a light, triangle, wheel, flower, stone, etc.) in front of you. It should be an anchor that connects you with the Divine.

Affirmation
Thy will be done.

44

MUDRA OF THE INNER SELF

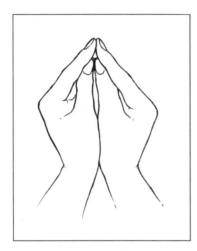

Place together the tips of your index, middle, ring, and little fingers and the balls of your hands. Put the thumbs next to each other. Like a "street," they lead to the fingertips of the little fingers, which they touch. An empty space, through which light shimmers, is formed beneath the tips of the little fingers. This opening characterises the power of the heart through divine wisdom. This opening is different for every human being. Sophie Rodelli, who has been intensely involved with hand exercises and positions for many years, says: "This mudra symbolises the inner nature of the human being, which is concealed by physical power – but is aired at times through joy or suffering, or guided through the secret school by the inner human being."[17]

First hold your hands in this position in front of your forehead, and look through the opening, without blinking, as long as you can. Then lower your arms and hold the mudra an inch or so beneath your chin for a while. Your hands will automatically be at the spot where the place of the soul lies, according to the ancient mysteries, and they form a temple around it. Now pay attention to your breathing. With every exhalation,

[17] Sofie Rodelli, *Handübungen als Heilgymnastik* (Munich, 1961), p. 73.

very gently whisper "Hoooo" and let yourself be carried through the little opening into infinity – into the great mystery.

When we hold this mudra while sitting in the meditation position with crossed legs, many triangles are formed with our body parts: beginning with the little space between the fingers; above the hands, arms, legs, and the entire body posture. The triangle is the symbol of the Divine, and our body now expresses this through its posture in a number of ways. This mudra is a prayer without words – a silent meditation, a devotion to the Divine.

With this mudra, we enter the realm of the unfathomable, the Divine. It is the only mudra that I dared to describe on a holy Sunday while rewriting the manuscript. Moreover, after meditating on this mudra today, I "coincidentally" came across a poem by Hermann Hesse:

We live on in form and illusion
And only sense in days of suffering
The eternal changeless existence
Of which dark dreams tell us.

We are delighted at deceit and delusion,
We are like blind men without a guide,
In time and space we anxiously seek
What can only be found in eternity.

We hope for redemption and salvation
In the unreal offerings of dreams –
Since we are gods and take part
In the very beginnings of Creation.[18]

---

[18] Hermann Hesse, *Traumgeschenk,* p. 311, trans. from German.

45

LOTUS MUDRA

(Symbol of purity)

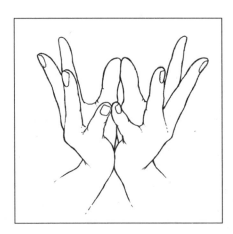

Place both hands in front of your chest so that only the edges of your hands and pads of your fingers touch each other: This is the bud of the lotus flower. Now open your hands, but maintain the contact between the tips of the little fingers and the outer edges of your thumbs. Spread the other fingers open as wide as possible. After four deep breaths, close both hands back into a bud, place the finger-nails of the fingers of both hands on top of each other; now join the backs of the fingers, the backs of the hands, and let your hands hang down relaxed for a while. In the same way, bring your hands back into the bud and the open flower. Repeat a number of times.

This mudra belongs to the heart chakra and is the symbol for purity. Love lives in the heart, together with goodwill, affection, and communication. We are meant to keep it pure and give it unconditionally, like an open flower that holds its chalice open for the insects. It is their nourishment and gives them warmth on cold nights. In turn, the insects pollinate it and help it fulfil the purpose of its existence. We are connected with our fellow human beings in more or less the same way – in both the good sense and the bad – and dependent upon them. However, the open flower has another message waiting for us. It opens to the sun, the divine principle, and lets itself be given whatever it needs; and it is given in abundance – it receives much more than it "needs." We enjoy blossoming flowers because they bear joy, the divine countenance, within themselves, and exude it to us.

Do this mudra when you feel drained, exploited, misunderstood, or lonely. Open yourself to the divine force and receive whatever you need – and much more.

Imagine the bud of a lotus flower (or a water lily) in your heart. Every time you inhale, the flower opens a bit more – until it finally is completely open and can absorb the full sunlight into itself. It lets itself be filled with light, lightness, warmth, love, desire, and joy.

Affirmation
I open myself to nature; I open myself to the good that exists in every human being; and I open myself to the Divine so that I will be richly blessed.

46

ABHAYA MUDRA

(Gesture for promising protection)

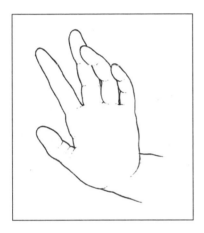

Raise your right hand to chest level with the palm facing forward. Place your left hand on your left thigh, in your lap, or on your heart.

We see this gesture in many depictions of deities. It promises the believer protection and freedom from fear. It also shows the strength of the respective deity.

We must remember that fear or fright are basically signs of weakness. The Chinese Five Element Theory shows that, among other things, a weakness in the fire element creates a fear of others, in the wood element it creates a fear of being defined through others; in the metal element it creates a fear of too little or too much distance (loneliness); in the earth and water elements it creates a fear of challenges and life in general. Fear has infinitely many faces, but its cause is always weakness. The greatest commandment of the yogis is nonviolence. The stronger a person is, which also includes strength on the mental-emotional level, the more he or she will be able to live nonviolence, since a strong person is rarely attacked. Many people are weakened as a result of inner conflicts, because of a certain lack of unity within themselves. These inner battles are then carried out in the outside world by attracting the appropriate battle partner. We must keep all of this in mind when we seek refuge in this mudra. However, just doing the mudra does not solve the problem. Since coming to terms with these negative patterns of the soul is a long process of transformation, together with the recommended visualisation, this mudra may help initially in frightening situations.

Imagine a silver or golden funnel in your mind. While *inhaling,* divine light (courage, goodwill, confidence) flows through the funnel into your head. From there, it flows on into your body. Let yourself be filled with it. While *exhaling,* the light flows back out through your right hand and you direct it toward the respective person or thing that you must confront. Perhaps you would like to reach more than one person with it – go ahead and do whatever comes to you naturally. Do this meditation more frequently for a person or thing that causes you concern, and let yourself be surprised by the positive results!

Affirmation
I believe in the good in this human being (or in this thing) and the good will be revealed to me.

47

VARADA MUDRA

(Gesture of granting wishes or mercy)

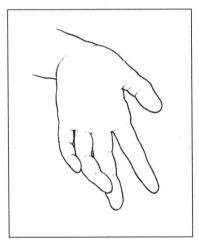

Point the left hand downward and turn the palm to the front. Place the right hand on your lap or thigh.

This mudra is a preferred gesture in the depiction of Hindu gods. As the name indicates, this is a matter of forgiveness and mercy. Moreover, the believers hope that God will bless them richly – fulfil their wishes. This is aptly expressed. Someone who gives will be forgiven, someone who forgives will be richly blessed. Forgiveness always also means being able to forgive yourself. To forgive yourself and others is certainly the most difficult thing one can ask of a person. But it is truly the most wonderful thing when we succeed at it. The forgiving open hand is then filled with new riches, both inner and outer. I speak from experience here and can warmly recommend the "art of forgiveness" to you. Perhaps it may be difficult for you at first; if so, ask the divine force that lives within you for help.

It is also important to know that the intensive work of forgiveness should not be done throughout the entire year – that would wear us down too much. But it fits wonderfully into a spring or autumn detoxification programme.

The saying, "Let's bury it," gets to the main issue of forgiveness, and nature demonstrates how and why every autumn. If the seeds are not put under the soil, then no new plants would grow. If we cannot bury our past, this may burden us so much that we become ill; it will also obstruct our inner development.

Imagine that you have an object in front of you that belongs to the person who is involved with your need for forgiveness. With each exhalation, blow your negative feelings onto and into this object. In conclusion, put the object in a package and bury it in a place that has a special meaning for you. You can imagine this or you can do it as a ritual and actually bury the negativity in the ground.

Perhaps you may later frequently visit this place in your mind and send the respective person good thoughts. Since no healthy and happy human being will want to hurt another, the people who have tormented us are in particular need of our prayers. You don't have to be a saint to do this – but you will become "healed and whole" if you practise it now and then.

Affirmation

I forgive myself for all the wrong things that I have done and/or said.
I forgive you for all the wrong things that you
have ever done and/or said.

48

BHUMISPARSHA MUDRA

(Gesture of enlightenment, or gesture of calling witnesses)

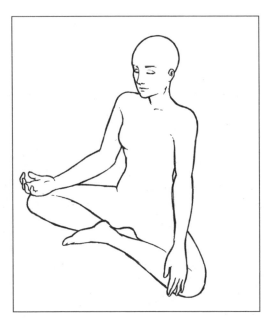

Point the left hand down to the earth and let your fingers touch the ground. Let the right hand point upward to Heaven, like an open flower.

Buddha, like Jesus, was tempted by evil before he began proclaiming his teachings, but both were successful in resisting it. Mara, god of sensual desires, attempted to talk Buddha into believing that he was not even entitled to the tiny bit of earth where he sat in meditation. Then Buddha touched the ground with the fingers of his right hand and swore he would bear witness that he was indeed quite entitled to remain on Earth because of his many good deeds. This legend shows how important it is for people to first fulfil their earthly obligations if they want to achieve enlightenment.

If we are aware that cosmic consciousness in all its forms manifests itself in everything and everyone around us, that we are connected with everything through our individual consciousness, then the first commandment of all great religions becomes clear to us. Love yourself and love the world around you – you and the world around you are one – we are all part of the greater whole – what is on the inside is on the outside – the whole is greater than the sum of its parts – the greatest lives within the smallest. We will never be able to completely fathom the entire dimensions of this power, and this is also good.

Simply look at an object or being (stone, plant, animal, etc.). While *inhaling,* absorb its energy; while *exhaling,* give it your energy. Each breath is like a band, and the connection becomes denser and denser until you merge with it. You can connect with cosmic consciousness in this way, and it will show you the path to eternal unity.

Affirmation
Connected with cosmic consciousness, I feel myself guided, protected, supported, and upheld on my path in life.

49

DHARMACHAKRA MUDRA

(Gesture of turning the wheel)

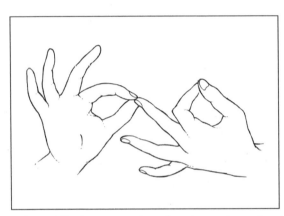

Raise both hands in front of your chest with your right hand somewhat higher than the left. Join the thumbs and index fingers of each hand. The palm of your left hand faces your heart, and the back of your right hand faces your body. The left middle finger touches the place where the thumb and index finger of the right hand form a closed circle.

Before you continue to read, pause for a moment and try the Dharmachakra Mudra. While forming it, breathe very deeply, slowly, and finely; focus on how the three fingertips are touching each other. How do you feel? It is possible for you to notice a change in your mood or not?

The hands form two wheels. In Hindu mythology, the wheel embodies completion or the wheel of life that guides us through a diversity of experiences. But there are two wheels here, and this indicates the teaching of reincarnation. The left middle finger (Saturn) represents the transition from this world into the next – from death and birth.

For me, this mudra has an additional, very special meaning. The left hand, which points to my heart, symbolises my inner world; the right hand indicates my surrounding world. The inside and outside must be in harmony. Otherwise, my energy is not balanced, and I am not happy. This means, for example, that I must make my contribution to society, that I must fulfil my duties. Only then can I go off into peace and silence. But it is also important that I allow myself enough time for self-communion, from which I draw new strength and wisdom. This mudra also draws attention to the fact of eternal change. A guiding principle that applies to both the good times and the bad times says: *This too shall pass.* If we remember this, we are already a little bit closer to inner serenity, even-mindedness, and harmony.

Visualise a figure of light, your higher self, and ask it to wisely guide you through the ups and downs of life. You can ask it *anything.* Then remain in silence for a while afterward and listen – perhaps the figure of light also has something to say to you.

Affirmation
*With a grateful heart, I entrust my being to my higher self,
who knows what is best for me.*

VAJRAPRADAMA MUDRA

(Gesture of unshakable trust)

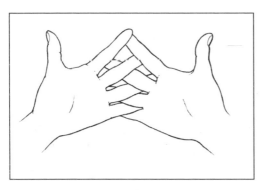

Cross the fingers of both hands in front of your chest. Solid fundamental trust is the basis for healthy self-confidence. We experience times when we think we can deal with whatever comes our way; and there are times when we doubt ourselves, we feel insecure and think ourselves not capable of handling anything that happens. When we take a closer look at things, we notice how important inner strength is for our self-confidence. When we are weakened, no matter on what level (physical, mental, emotional), then insecurity sneaks in. We can build up our inner strength with specific mudras, physical exercises, and breathing exercises (see page 43).

Furthermore, I have noticed that I begin to doubt and brood or feel insecure when I lose my connection with cosmic consciousness. Isn't it wonderful to know that we are just one single thought away from it and can overcome this distance at any time? Cosmic consciousness, or the Divine, is always there – but where are we? This perception has changed my entire life.

To always be reminded of this fact, you can place an object – something like a talisman – in your pocket, or on your desk/workstation.

At the beginning of the meditation, formulate your question or request in precise and clear terms, either out loud or quietly. Then give thanks for the directions that are given to you. For the rest of the meditation, simply be still and direct your attention to your breathing.

Affirmation
I am a creation of the greatest omnipotence, whose strength and power lovingly support me at all times.

51

NAGA MUDRA

(Naga, the snake goddess, symbolises supernatural strength, wisdom, shrewdness, and potency)

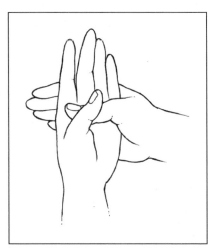

Cross your hands in front of your chest, and also cross your thumbs over each other. This gesture is sometimes called "the mudra of deeper insight." Even when we take the spiritual path, we will encounter worldly challenges time and time again. Only by working through these challenges do we progress on the path; and only so can we fulfil the purpose of our lives. This is why the Naga Mudra can be successfully used to solve everyday problems. Answers can also be expected to questions about decisions that must be made, the meaning of a specific matter, the future, and the spiritual path. When we need to know something, then we will also know it at the right time. But we must question and listen.

Blazing fire is a powerful element. It warms, moves, and activates us. This is why visualisations of fire always set something in motion, develop strength, and pleasantly relieve tensions. When we mentally kindle the fire in our pelvic floor, this will not only give us strength, but also light. We can carry this light with us like a torch, and it will show us the way.

With your powers of imagination, kindle a fire in your pelvic floor. While *inhaling,* let the flames flicker high upward so you encounter the world with a fiery heart. Let the flames continue to rise higher so you have a bright, clear head. Your breaths are deep and powerful at the beginning; with time, they become slow, fine, and flowing. Each inhalation causes you to sit straighter, both inwardly and outwardly, as if you were being pulled upward. While *exhaling,* hold onto your new size but let go of every inner tension. Stay in the stillness for a while. First ask your questions, and then listen inside yourself.

Affirmation
All my senses are focused on the Divine, and I thankfully accept its wise advice and its deeds.

52

PUSHPAPUTA MUDRA

(A handful of flowers)

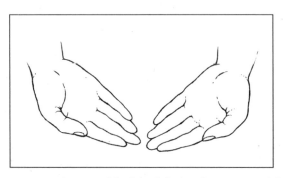

Place your hands like empty bowls on your thighs. Let your fingers rest next to each other in a relaxed way, with the thumbs against the outer edge of the index finger.

The focus here is openness and accep-
tance. What wealth does life (or the universe) have waiting for us? How often do we pass it by without paying any attention? How often are we outwardly or inwardly closed to a new opportunity?

How often do we ignore the gentle hints from the universe until we need the blows of fate to get back on the right track? We can be spared all this if we remain open. One reason why we close ourselves – in addition to apathy – is fear. But whatever is bad cannot get to us and affect us if we strive for a pure heart. This is a law of the cosmos. We can only attract what also has an equivalent within us. This is why mental-emotional hygiene is so important. We can hardly avoid the negative feelings that occasionally arise within us, but we can also come to terms with them and transform them at any time. This is part of the maturation process.

The Pushpaputa Mudra expresses this openness. Only with open hands can we enrich the world, and only with an open mind and open soul can we receive what cosmic consciousness gives us.

Your two hands are like open flowers. Imagine another flower on top of your head. While *inhaling,* golden rays come from a cosmos that embodies love, warmth, joy, and peace. Through the open flowers, they flow into your innermost self. Then let yourself be filled (take a pause in your breathing for a moment) and radiate this wealth through your heart into the world while *exhaling.*

Affirmation
I open myself to divine joy (or healing power, light, love, etc.), let myself be filled by it. I radiate it into the world through my heart.

THE MUDRAS OF
HATHA YOGA

*W*e find the first written records of the mudras of Hatha Yoga in the *Hatha Yoga Pradipika* (*Pradipika* means the "little lamp of yoga") and in the *Gheranda Samita* (the collected teachings of the sage Gheranda). Ten mudras are discussed in the first work and 15 more in the second, making a total of 25 mudras. According to these writings, the effects of the mudras extend from healing everyday complaints to maintaining youthful freshness at a ripe old age, to even determining one's own day of death. However, many yoga masters think that these promises should not be taken too literally. They say these are superficial explanations for non-initiates. The deeper aspects of the mudras are only revealed to those who seriously practise them through the guidance of a teacher.

Classical mudras are mainly used for awakening kundalini, experiencing states of expanded consciousness, or achieving enlightenment. Since such practises are like a tightrope walk and accordingly dangerous, they can only be learned with an experienced teacher. The way in which I use the mudras in daily life and present them here, they primarily serve the health of body, mind, and soul. This is reason enough for me to practise them.

Swami Satyananda Saraswati, a recognised Hindu yoga master, was the first to describe them so that even we normal mortals can do them. He also gives the advice of practicing the mudras in combination with body postures (asanas) and breathing exercises (pranayamas) since this will considerably intensify the body and breathing work. Mudras are also the ideal preparation for meditation. Today, other directions such as Power Yoga and Kundalini Yoga, agree with his opinion.

I will first present the mudras that are practised in the seated meditation position and then a mudra sequence.

Exercises in the Seated Meditation Position

JNANA MUDRA AND CHIN MUDRA

(Gesture of knowledge and gesture of wisdom)

The only hand mudra mentioned in Hatha Yoga is found on page 3.
- Assume the seated meditation posture and hold this mudra as described.

BHUCHARI MUDRA

(The gaze into the void)

- Assume the seated meditation posture in front of a white wall (with your eyes looking at the wall).
- Place the thumb of your right hand between your nose and upper lip.
- Stare at your little finger.
- After a short while, lower your hand and continue to look at the place where the little finger had been.
- Concentrate as long as possible on this spot and think of nothing else.

Effect: Promotes memory and concentration and calms the mind.

SHAMBAVI MUDRA

(Glance directed upward between the eyebrows)

- Assume seated meditation posture and form the Chin or Jnana Mudra with the hands (see page 139).
- Direct your gaze inward and upward, as if you wanted to look at the centre of your forehead.
- Calm your thoughts; don't think of anything; or just observe your breathing.
- End the mudra as soon as your eyes get tired.

Effect: I encountered this mudra at Mental Training.[19] It has also been tested and found to have a very calming and stress-reducing effect. It is considered one of the most highly developed techniques of yoga. With this mudra, we are said to transcend the mental world and are able to enter into the realm of highest consciousness.

AGOCHARI MUDRA

(Gaze at the tip of the nose)

- Assume the seated meditation posture, form the Jnana or Chin Mudra with your hands (see page 139).
- Focus your eyes on the tip of your nose.
- As soon as your eyes get tired, end the mudra.

Effect: This mudra promotes concentration, calms the nervous system, and stimulates the root chakra.

---

[19] Gerhard H. Eggetsberger, *Power für den ganzen Tag* (Wien, 1995), p. 40.

AKASHI MUDRA

(The consciousness of inner space – tongue on the gums)

- Assume the seated meditation posture.
- Place the thumbs of both hands on the pad of your middle finger of the respective hand.
- Raise your chin a bit and direct your eyes upward to the centre of the forehead.
- Roll your tongue backward and place the tip on the gums.
- Observe the four phases of breathing (inhalation, extended pause, exhalation, extended pause).

Effect: This is another mudra that I have encountered in Western mental techniques. It quickly brings us into a light trance, activates the brain activity, calms the emotions, and creates an inner balance. The tongue position has a positive influence on the limbic system, which is responsible for our feelings and moods. It also supports the integration of both brain hemispheres. In relation to the meridian system, the tongue on the gums activates important meridians. As a result, these experience an energy lock and charge themselves more intensely. It is worthwhile to practise this mudra a few minutes a day for a number of weeks.

BHUJANGANI MUDRA

(Snake breathing)

- Assume the seated meditation posture and hold your hands in Mudra Number 8 (see page 74).
- Now swallow the air as if slurping water, and direct it to your abdomen.

- Arch your abdomen in a relaxed way and hold the air for a moment in this area.
- Let the air back out again by belching.
- It is sufficient to do this exercise 3 to 5 times in a row.

Effect: This mudra strengthens the abdomen, eliminates gases, has a cleansing effect on the digestive tract, and makes stomach complaints disappear.

KAKI MUDRA

(Raven beak)

- Assume the seated meditation posture.
- Shape your lips so they form an "O."
- Focus your eyes on the tip of your nose.
- Now inhale slowly and thoroughly through your mouth.
- Now close your mouth and hold your breath for about 10 seconds.
- Then exhale very slowly through the nose.
- Repeat 10 to 30 times.

Effect: The Kaki Mudra has a cleansing effect on the mouth, gums, and the entire upper digestive tract, from the stomach far into the intestines. Accordingly, it also causes the skin to become more pure. In addition, it has a calming effect on the autonomous nervous system. It also improves the sense of taste for sweet, salty, sour, and bitter. And finally, it stimulates the secretion of saliva and has a cooling effect.

YONI MUDRA

(Seal of the inner source)

- Assume the seated meditation posture and now breathe slowly, rhythmically, and deeply.
- Hold your breath and close your ears with your thumbs, the eyes with your index fingers, and the nostrils with your middle fingers. Place the ring fingers on your lips and the little fingers beneath them to close your mouth.
- Take the middle finger from your nose and slowly exhale. Leave the other fingers where they are.
- Inhale and then close the nostrils again.
- Hold your breath and feel your way into the silence.
- Take the middle finger away again and exhale.
- Repeat a number of times.

Effect: A wonderful silence arises and all the sensory organs become sensitised. This also achieves a quick and deliberate disconnection from outer influences.

SHANTI MUDRA

(The mudra of peace)

- Assume the seated meditation posture. Close your eyes and place your hands in your lap.
- Exhale completely. Concentrate on your root chakra (see Appendix D) and do the Maha Bandha (see page 172).
- Hold your breath for several seconds.
- While inhaling, release the Maha Bandha. When the lungs

are filled with air and the body arches slightly, place your hands on your stomach (solar plexus chakra), the sternum (heart chakra), and forehead (forehead chakra).

- Now spread your arms widely and concentrate on your crown chakra.
- Repeat a number of times.

Effect: Deepens the breathing. A feeling of peace may arise. This mudra also kindles the vital energy in the root chakra, distributes it throughout the entire body, and therefore helps us achieve inner strength, personal magnetism, and health, says Swami Satyananda Saraswati. You can associate an additional, very lovely spiritual aspect with this mudra when you imagine the power that rises from your root chakra to be the energy of peace. It fills your body, your soul, and your mind. By spreading your arms, you send vital energy out into the world – it becomes a gesture of blessing.

MAHA BANDHA

The so-called bandhas (lock exercises) are also associated with the mudras in classical yoga.

- Assume the seated meditation posture. Now exhale well. At the same time, press your hands onto your thighs and tighten the musculature around the perineum (PC) by tensing the bladder and the sphincter muscles at the same time, as if you wanted to hold back feces and urine (Mula Bandha). In ordinary exercise this is call the Kegel exercise.
- Then pull in the abdominal wall (Uddiyana Bandha).
- And press the chin onto the larynx (Jalandhara Bandha).

- After a few seconds, release every tension, raise the chin, and inhale deeply.
- Repeat a number of times.

Effect: The Maha Bandha can be used for a weak bladder, hemorrhoids, constipation, descended organs, weak digestion, flat breathing, or neck tension; it has a preventive effect on these symptoms or diseases. The brain energy is also activated by the contractions of the bandha. I usually practise the Maha Bandha before meditation, which helps me go into a deeper state more quickly. It may lead to a light trance, which can sometimes be quite pleasant.

PART THREE

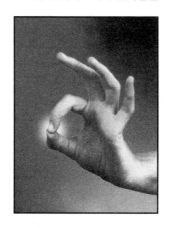

Practical

Applications

MUDRA EXERCISES

*A*s mentioned earlier, a few of the body positions in Hatha Yoga are also called mudras. I have combined these with other yoga exercises and put together a beneficial, meaningful series of exercises. I offer it as an additional approach, so you can use it, or not, in keeping with your needs. If yes, then slowly speak the affirmation given at the end of the exercise 1 to 3 times, either after or during the exercise, in your own breathing rhythm.

You can consider this series of exercises to be preparation for meditation or you can practise them after meditation. Particularly when you have been sitting for a longer period of time, the exercises are an absolute relief. They can also be done separate from the meditation period in your morning or evening yoga ritual. Since the effect is considerably dependent upon the thoughts and feelings that come during the practise, I have included an affirmation with each exercise.

LIMBER-UP AND WARM-UP EXERCISE

- Form the hands into Atmanjali (Mudra Number 42).

- At first, remain calm, standing for several breaths, while you collect yourself in the heart centre.

- *Inhale:* Stretch your arms upward.

- *Exhale:* Bring your hands back to your chest, bend your knees and squat down.

- *Inhale:* Come back up, and stretch your arms upward.

- *Exhale.*

- Repeat a number of times.

Affirmation
I connect myself with the powers of Heaven and Earth.

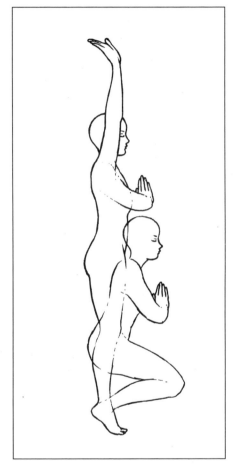

Effect: Calms and collects the mind; warms up the body.

THE MESSAGE OF SHIVA

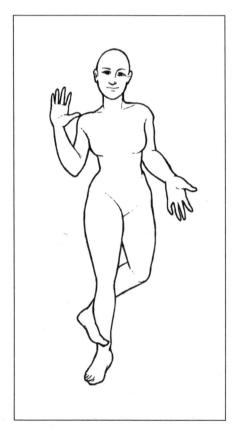

- Stand on the right leg; bend the left leg.

- Form your right hand into the gesture to turn away fear (Mudra Number 46) and form the gesture of mercy (Mudra Number 47) with the left hand.

- Remain in this position for 10 breaths.

- Change the leg position and remain in this pose for another ten breaths.

Affirmation
I feel protected and supported by the heavenly powers and show myself as having goodwill and mercy toward every fellow being.

Effect: Strengthens inner stability and self-assurance. Gives us the courage to show the goodness of our hearts.

YOGA MUDRA

(Seal of unity)

So that you can sit comfortably and bend forward as far as possible, it may be necessary to place a thick, stable cushion beneath your buttocks.

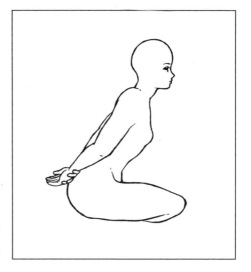

- Sit with your legs crossed, hands on your back, with one hand encircling the other.

- *Inhale:* The consciousness travels from the root chakra to the forehead chakra.

- Hold breath: Keep concentrating on the forehead chakra for several seconds.

- *Exhale:* Bend forward and direct your consciousness from the forehead chakra back down to your root chakra.

- Hold breath: Keep concentrating on the root chakra for several seconds.

- *Inhale:* Sit up straight and direct the consciousness from the root chakra to the forehead chakra again.

- *Exhale.*

- Repeat 6 times until it becomes a flowing movement.

- Now cross your legs the other way, encircle the other hand, and repeat the whole exercise again 6 times.

Affirmation
With thanks and praise, I accept what the universe has waiting for me.

Effect: This mudra "massages" the lower abdominal organs, which are responsible for numerous complaints, such as digestive disorders, constipation, menstrual complaints, and bladder problems. The individual vertebra are separated from each other, whereby the spinal nerves that emerge from the vertebra are gently stretched and stimulated. These nerves connect the entire body with the brain so this vitalisation has an effect on overall health. The solar plexus chakra, which is considered one of the most important sources of energy, is stimulated to a special degree. The Yoga Mudra also helps reduce pent-up aggravation and tension, giving a person inner repose and peace. It makes the nadis, the subtle energy channels, permeable so that the elemental force from the root chakra can rise upward.

TWIST IN THE SEATED MEDITATION POSTURE

- Place left hand on right knee, and stretch your right arm to the back.

- *Inhale* and turn to the right while doing so.

- Press your right shoulder as far as possible to the back and look over your shoulder.

- Remain in the twist for 15 breaths.

- *Exhale* and return to the middle while doing so.

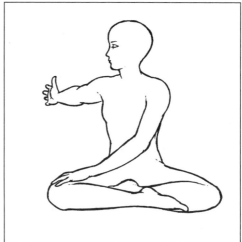

- Raise your arms upward, stretch vigorously, and twist to the other side. The upward twist at the conclusion is very important.

- Change your leg position, twist to both sides again, then stretch upward through the middle a number of times.

Affirmation
In the form of a spiral, my path leads to the divine goal where joy and peace rule.

Effect: This massages the ganglia and organs; it strengthens the nervous system, liver, spleen, pancreas, and gallbladder; it stimulates the metabolism in the vertebra; and it stretches and squeezes the ligaments and muscles along the spinal column.

SIDE STRETCH

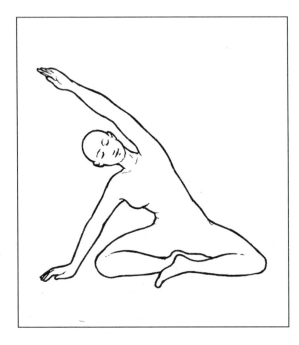

- Assume the seated meditation posture.

- Prop up one hand on each side.

- *Inhale:* Lift your right arm and stretch vigorously upward.

- Hold breath: Pull your arm to the left.

- *Exhale:* Lower arm to side and prop up your hand again.

- Repeat six times; then practise on the other side.

- Change your leg position, then bend again on both sides.

Affirmation
*I open myself to what is beautiful and good and everything that
I need for my spiritual journey.*

Effect: Supports effect of the previous exercise.

TADAGI MUDRA

(Pond seal)

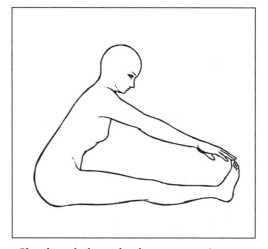

- Assume an upright seated posture with legs extended; place your fingers on your toes, and draw in your chin somewhat.

- *Inhale:* Arch the abdominal wall outward as far as possible.

- Hold your breath for a few seconds, and then concentrate on the solar plexus chakra. Slowly exhale and relax your entire body.

- Inhale and exhale in a relaxed way one more time, then repeat the entire exercise ten times.

Affirmation
With a fiery torch, I encounter the challenges of life.

Effect: An excellent exercise for all the organs, especially for the stomach, lungs, and intestines.

MAHA MUDRA

(Large seal)

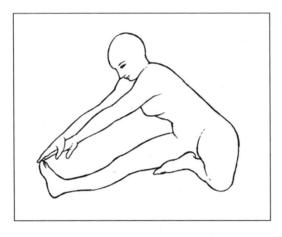

- Sit with spread and extended legs. Place your left foot on your right thigh and then touch your fingers to your toes or leg. Draw your chin in vigorously and keep your back straight (don't stoop).

- Now do the Maha Bandha (see page 171) three times.

- And then remain in this position for 20 more breaths.

- In conclusion, bend your leg, hug it, and relax. Place your forehead on the knee and rest for 10 breaths.

- Straighten up again, change your leg position, and practise on the other side.

Affirmation

My inner powers develop and fulfil me.

Effect: This mudra causes the most important energy channels to flow better, and it stimulates the organs of the abdomen and pelvis.

PASCIMOTTANASANA

(Backstretch)

Remain completely relaxed in the forward bend for a number of breaths. Let your upper body be supported by your legs, and allow your head to hang down in a relaxed way.

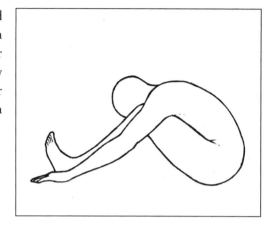

Affirmation
I feel myself wonderfully supported by the powers of good.

Effect: The blood circulation in the pelvis is intensified; repose, relaxation, and a sense of being centred arise. This is the position of self-communion.

ARDHA CAKRASANA

(Bridge)

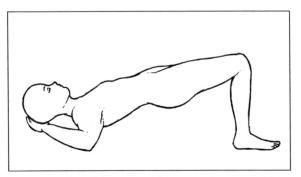

- Lay on your back with feet propped up at hip's width.

- *Inhale:* Raise the buttocks and the back.

- Hold breath: Vigorously contract the anal sphincter and tense the musculature of the pelvic floor (Ashwini Mudra).

- *Exhale* and once again let go of the tension.

- Repeat a number of times and then lower your back while exhaling.

Affirmation

My heart's bridge leads from time into eternity.

Effect: Strengthens and firms the outer and inner muscles in area of anus and entire pelvic floor. Prevents atony (slackness) of outer anal sphincter, from which many older people suffer.

PASHINI MUDRA

(Noose seal: simplified form)

- Draw your knees to the chest, wrap your arms under the hollow of your knees, and place your palms on the ears.

- Hold (a) the position for 10 breaths and then remain in the fetus position (b) for a few seconds.

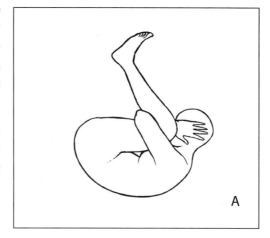

A

Affirmation
Repose and peace fill me completely.

Effect: Calms the nerves and regulates the thyroid gland.

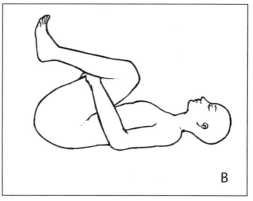

B

VIPARITA KARANI MUDRA

(Half-candle)

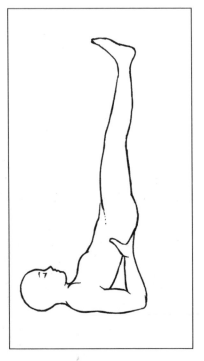

- Lie in a supine position, with your legs propped up at hip's distance.

- *Inhale:* Bring knees to chest and then bring your legs into the vertical position. Support the pelvis with your hands.

- During the first breath, concentrate on the solar plexus chakra; during the second, on the heart chakra; during the third, on the throat chakra; during the forth, on the solar plexus chakra again, and so on.

- Hold the position for 12 to 36 breaths.

- *Exhale:* Bend knees and bring to forehead; then carefully and slowly return to the floor so you are lying on your back.

Affirmation
In my depths lives the Highest.

Effect: Improves blood circulation in the entire body and has a cleansing effect on the lungs, bladder, and intestines.

KARTARI MUDRA

(Resting position)

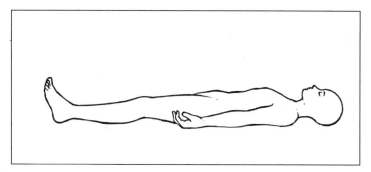

- Lie in a supine position; place your hands next to your body or on your abdomen, with the right hand on top of the left.

- Now inhale deeply and arch the abdominal wall. As soon as the abdomen is full, slide your hands to your ribs and expand this region. When your ribs are spread as much as possible, slide your hands to the collarbone and raise the area above the chest.

- Slowly exhale and repeat the process a number of times.

With each exhalation, let yourself become heavier and heavier. Release your weight to the supporting floor. While *inhaling,* let yourself be filled with lightness and light; while *exhaling,* let go of everything heavy and dark within you. At the close, you are full of light, freedom, peace, and joy.

Effect: Improves and deepens breathing, regenerates the autonomic nervous system (organ activity), and relaxes the entire body.

HOW TO CREATE
YOUR OWN MUDRA

*O*nce you have studied this book and become thoroughly acquainted with the energies of your hands, you can also create your own mudra.

- When you develop a mudra, the proper frame of mind and respect are important preconditions for success.

- Study the qualities of the individual fingers and choose the respective posture.

- In positive wording, formulate the result or goal that you want to achieve through the mudra. Use the present tense.

- Speak the sentence at least three times out loud, and slowly in the rhythm of your breath.

- Visualise precisely how the result or goal will look.

- Try to already feel how it is when the result occurs.

- Place the mudra under the protection of the divine forces, a saint, or an angel whom you revere in particular.

- Wish for the result with great fervour, but remain completely patient and serene.

WHAT A MUDRA
CANNOT DO

*I*n this book, there was a lot of talk about healing in both a physical as well as a mental and emotional way. But what if this doesn't happen? There may be various reasons responsible for this. Perhaps you are impatient. You now know that – particularly in chronic diseases that have often slumbered in the body for many years before they erupted – a mudra must be held every day for a number of weeks or months until the effect arises. It is also possible that thoughts, feelings, and/or moods do not let us become healthy. Health also means inner peace, and we can only have this when we live in peace with our surrounding world as well. It is also possible that we live in discontentment with our inner forces. Perhaps you can lovingly work on these problems and eliminate or transform whatever is destructive.

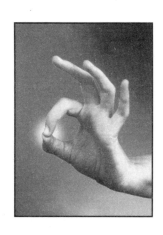

Appendices

APPENDIX A: NUTRITION

*M*udra experts, such as Keshav Dev and Kim da Silva, recommend paying attention to nutrition simultaneously with practising the mudras. The ancient yogis also knew this. The extent to which the body fluids (blood, lymph) are permeable for both the physical and the subtle energies is largely dependent upon how much waste material is in the body. Our waste material is created based on our choice of foods. For example, one of my acquaintances, who for years has required medication to treat high blood pressure (deposits in the blood vessels can be the cause of high blood pressure), suddenly could not tolerate the medication anymore. Despite great concern on the part of the physician, he reduced the dosage to a minimum; this made my friend feel much better and his blood pressure remained normal. How did this happen? His wife changed his diet and, after a few months of the new diet, he reacted in this way because the deposits in the blood vessels had been reduced.

For many years now, I have been intensely interested in nutrition. In the days when I worked assisting senior citizens, during house visits I made a little game of looking at the people at the door and guessing all the things that would be in their kitchens. I was rarely wrong.

If I were to start eating like most people, asthma and allergies would return within a short period of time. But the truth is that my allergies have been gone since 1985, and have never returned after I did a 9-day lemon juice treatment. This is my current diet:

Upon arising: I drink a glass of water.

Breakfast: Green tea or herb tea, wholegrain bread with butter or curd (kefir) cheese and sprouts and a piece of cheese.

Lunch: Salad or steamed vegetables, legumes, and a grain or potato dish.

Dinner: As little as possible. For example, vegetable soup, bread, cheese, flake muesli with a banana.

Snacks: In the morning, water, tea, and fruit; in the afternoon, a cup of coffee with a little piece of chocolate or a few sweet biscuits.

I only eat meat or fish occasionally on the weekends. Too much meat obstructs my breathing and makes me aggressive; but an even more important reason is that I love animals and don't want to eat them. I have also eliminated milk, tomatoes, hot peppers, and kiwis from my diet because they intensify mucous congestion in the lungs and digestive tract.

One thing is for certain – you must design your own diet plan and adapt it to the needs of your body. Don't ask too much of yourself. It is better to use a bit of cleverness. I reduced my consumption of meat (my father was a butcher and meat was therefore the main thing on the menu at home) by asking myself every day: "Does it have to be meat or could I also satisfy my hunger and cravings with something vegetarian?" When I had a genuine desire for meat, then I enjoyed the meat. But I increasingly noticed that I could just as well eat something else. With time, I reduced my meat consumption to a minimum. Keep the powerful and intelligent elephants in mind – they are vegetarians.

I was also able to reduce my excessive consumption of black tea (the only addiction that I ever had) with a trick. I mixed it with green tea and constantly increased the proportion of green tea – until the black tea was no longer necessary. My herbal advisor, Elisabeth Steudler, swears by green tea since, like no other tea, it can truly be enjoyed at any time. It has a purifying effect, is good for the kidneys, urinary tract, and bladder, and has a preventive effect against cancer. One more tip: Wait until the boiling water has cooled down slightly before pouring it over the tea.

I also recommend the tea mixtures based on the Chinese Five Element Theory, which are available in health food stores and some pharmacies. In spring there is a tea mixture for the liver and gallbladder; in summer for the heart and circulation; in autumn for the stomach and pancreas; in late autumn for the lungs and large intestine; and in winter for the kidneys and bladder. Perhaps the following tips will be helpful to you.

- Particularly when it comes to oil, vinegar, sea salt, whole grains, and milk products – buy only first-class goods; whenever possible, also buy organic fruits and vegetables.

- In the morning, eat a great deal of fruit and drink a lot of fluids.

- At noon, eat primarily salads and foods containing protein.

- In the evening, eat as little as possible and primarily cooked vegetable and grain dishes.

- Eat simply and never mix more than three different kinds of vegetables.

- Chew well, eat slowly, and be in a good mood. Enjoy your food.

With these few reference points, you can put together a high-quality, sensible diet of whole foods – a diet that doesn't unnecessarily strain your system or fill it with waste materials, but builds it up, keeps your body healthy, refreshes your mind, and lifts your spirits.

There is no rule without an exception! If you don't have any physical complaints, you will certainly want to go out to eat occasionally. You certainly should do this and enjoy it!

APPENDIX B: THERE IS AN HERB FOR EVERY MALADY

*W*hen selecting herbs, Elisabeth Steudler and I have made sure that most of them come from our region (in Switzerland) and can be obtained in any pharmacy. You need to do the same thing in your area. Try to buy your herbs locally, or go to a good herb supplier. Only buy first-class goods, even if they cost considerably more. Today there are special measuring devices that can precisely analyze how much of the healing substances still exist in a dried herb. Planting, cultivation, harvesting, drying, and storage play a large role here. In order to preserve optimal quality, a great deal of expertise and care are necessary, and this has its price.

If you drink large quantities of herb teas, be sure to change to another variety as soon as an improvement occurs. The healing substances of many plants have the same effect as medications and can cause harm if taken excessively. Many herbs, such as an infusion of linden flowers (which can cause an outbreak of profuse sweating within a few minutes), have an immediate effect. The effect of other kinds of herbs can only be felt after hours or days.

Furthermore, you can create a mental connection with the respective herb by examining the nature of the plant. There are a great many wonderful books on this topic today, and you will find them in your metaphysical or health food stores. Don't hesitate to ask staff to recommend good books.

When you encounter plants while hiking, go ahead and discuss your concerns with them. Give yourself a magnifying glass for your next birthday so you can admire the great perfection of even the smallest plants – new worlds will be revealed to you. If you are ill and cannot spend time out in nature, plant photos can fulfil the same purpose. You can also use them to come into contact with the plant spirits, and this is what is important. Most plants are gentle and have a gentle effect – the tender touches are the ones that heal and help. They heal not only the body, but also the mind and soul, as proved by Edward Bach, the "father" of the Bach Flower Remedies. Open yourself to them today. It is exactly the right point in time.

Please respect the "useless" plants, for we don't know what they do! They are also creatures of the cosmic force and are certain to conceal very special secrets within themselves.

APPENDIX C: CHINESE FIVE ELEMENT THEORY

*F*or thousands of years, the energy of the body has played a significant role in traditional Chinese medicine. This healing method deals with energy in general and the energy of the individual organs in particular.

The Chinese observed that not every energy has the same quality. According to their respective qualities, they named the energies after the elements: wood, fire, earth, metal, water. Human beings also have within themselves the qualities of wood, for example; especially in the energy and/or in the meridians of the liver and gallbladder, but also in thinking and feeling. If this energy is weak, it shows in the corresponding organs, and also in our thoughts and moods. When we practise the mudras and their corresponding meditation images and affirmations, there is a positive effect on the respective energy and therefore also at the mental-emotional level.

Here are the qualities associated with the five elements:

Wood represents growth, a new beginning, stamina, and activity.

Fire represents individuality, heat, and generosity.

Earth represents a sense of being centred, digestion, change, and stability.

Metal represents clarity, cleanliness, and communication.

Water represents adaptability, sensitivity, repose, and the storage of life energies.

The following table will give you a brief survey of how the various qualities are related to the five elements. The bottom part of the table lists what strengthens or weakens an element or the associated organs. If necessary, you can also give some thought to what you could change or do in addition to the mudras in order to support healing, especially since some of the advice is quite pleasant. Laughing, singing, and dancing more often, or spending more time in the fresh air, aren't very frightening suggestions. When was the last time you saw a funny film or read a humourous book? When did you last dance, sing, or go to a sumptuous party?

Qualities of the Five Elements.

Qualities	Wood	Fire
Seasons	Spring	Summer
Direction of energy flow	Upward	In all directions
Associated meridians and organs	Liver, Gallbladder	Heart, Small intestine, Circulation, Triple warmer
Sensory organs	Eyes	Tongue
Body structures	Tendons, Articular cartilage, Nails, Hair	Blood vessels Body temperature
Taste	Sour	Bitter
Colour	Green	Red
Form	High, Cylindrical	Triangular, Pointed Sharp-edged
Emotions	Kindness, Control, Initiative, Anger	Joy, Openness Hatred
What strengthens the element?	Repose – especially lying down, Joy, Relaxation, Serenity, Positive visions of the future	Celebrating parties, Emotional warmth, Affection, Joy, Hiking or jogging, Dancing
What weakens the element?	Too much work, Too much sex, Too much travel, Too much food, Too much annoyance	Too little exercise, Emotional coldness, Loneliness, Excessive and lasting mental concentration.

Qualities of the Five Elements (continued).

Earth	Metal	Water
Late summer	Autumn	Winter
Downward	Inward	———
Spleen, Pancreas, Stomach	Lungs, Large intestine	Kidneys, Bladder
Mouth	Nose	Ears
Muscles	Skin	Bones
Sweet	Pungent	Salty
Yellow/brown	White	Blue/black
Flat, Square	Round	Wavy, Irregular
Repose, Being centred, Sympathy, Worry	Courage, Sense of order, Sadness, Resentment	Mercy, Adaptation, Contentment, Sense of security, Discontentment, Fear
Singing, A harmonious home, A sense of security, The right amount of good food in a harmonious atmosphere	Much movement in the outdoors, Breathing exercises, Having adequate time and space	Silent joy, Right amount of activity and rest, Healthy diet
Too much travel, Change of residence, Concern about others, Too much sweet, cold, or raw food	Lack of time, Too much constriction, Lack of contacts, Sadness, Mucous-forming foods	Lack of sleep, Irregular lifestyle, Fears, Continual stress, Noise, Too many lights, Excesses

APPENDIX D: SOME WORDS ABOUT THE CHAKRAS

Since there now is a great deal of literature on the topic of chakras, I will only give a very brief explanation of what they are and where they are located. The human being consists of many different energy levels, both physical and subtle. There are five energy vortexes along the spinal column. They move like wheels and have specific colours. There is an additional vortex in the area of the forehead and one more above the cranium. These are the so-called major chakras (there are also additional, minor chakras). The five chakras situated along the spinal column are associated with the five fingers. The chakras can be compared to transformers, as we know them from the field of electricity. They collect the energy that flows into the body, process and transform it, and distribute it again. The chakras are similar to the intersections of the energy paths, called *nadis,* which supply them with energy and carry it off again. In addition, they transform the frequencies into sensations that the human being understands: thinking and feeling. They make sure that the lack of energy is compensated for and the diverse energies are in the right place. They can also be called the organs of the energy body.

If consciousness is directed at one of the chakras for a period of time and on a frequent basis, this will activate its energy. This concept shouldn't be taken lightly, since too much energy can also be harmful. If you pay attention to the instructions given here, then only good things can happen. If the body is weakened, the chakras are usually also too weak in their

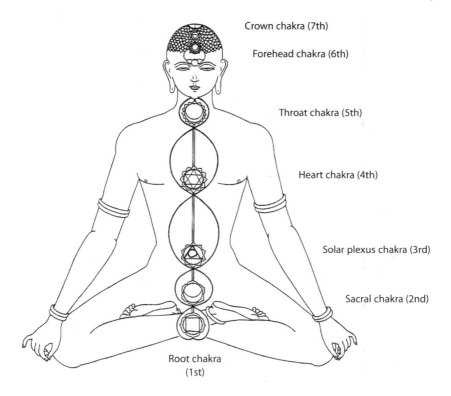

Crown chakra (7th)

Forehead chakra (6th)

Throat chakra (5th)

Heart chakra (4th)

Solar plexus chakra (3rd)

Sacral chakra (2nd)

Root chakra
(1st)

work and a bit more power won't be harmful.

If you would like to learn more about the chakras and how they work, I recommend the following book by Swami Sivananda Radha: *Kundalini Yoga for the West: A Foundation for Character Building, Courage and Awareness.*[20] As you can see in the table on page 206, the chakras and individual fingers also have character traits and talents associated with them.

---

[20] Sivananda, Radha, *Kundalini Yoga for the West: A Foundation for Character Building, Courage and Awareness* (Palo Alto, CA: Timeless Books, 1993).

The Chakras and the Corresponding Talents and Traits.

Chakra	Character Trait
Root chakra (1) (Muladhara)	Vitality, a sense of connection with Earth, basic trust, self-confidence, a sense of security in harmony with the laws of nature.
Sacral chakra (2) (Swadhisthana)	Survival of the species, sexuality, family, sociableness, creativity, solidarity with the surrounding world.
Solar plexus chakra (3) (Manipuraka)	Powers of imagination, visions of the future, desire for action, coming to terms with the past, decomposition; the inner fire that creates and destroys.
Heart chakra (4) (Anahata)	Love of life, joy, love, affection; source of unconditional, selfless love toward fellow human beings, every creature, every element, and the entire Creation.
Throat chakra (5) (Vishuddha)	Purity, ethics, knowledge, expanded consciousness, complete harmony.
Forehead chakra (6) (Ajna)	Dissolution of duality, regulation of all mental processes; rational thinking, intuition, inspiration, memory. Human beings see themselves as a unity here – consciousness, superconsciousness, and the subconscious mind flow together.
Crown chakra (7) (Sahasrara)	State of bliss, the individual consciousness connects with the cosmic consciousness here.

A CLOSING WORD

*W*ith joy and gratitude I end this book, for researching and writing it has brought me my own personal growth. I have gained new insights that will help me follow my path in life. The most important lesson was probably the continuously new development of *trust,* for as I began with the research, I "coincidentally" became acquainted with people who were scientifically and/or practically involved with the mudras and had also been using them successfully for years. My questions were always answered. I am telling you this to encourage you. I am not one bit better or more than you are – and if help was given to me, then help will also be there for you in every life situation.

Having trust in the Divine isn't just there for most of us. Perhaps you are similar to me, which means that you must – just like me – have to work on this basic trust thing time and time again. In doing so, I have found the following approaches to be particularly helpful. Go into silence as much as possible – even a few minutes are enough. Take everything seriously if it makes you feel discontented or unhappy, and *persistently* seek a solution. Every lack of health or joy that we feel because our relationships, our work, or our lives are not satisfactory has a special significance. It is an obstacle that must be overcome, which means we will work on this challenge if we wish to progress on our path in life.

We can approach our tasks in life with gnashing teeth or a playful flair. And the more serious the matter is, the more the lightness of *humour* can help us through it. Humour can lift us over the biggest stumbling blocks. Perhaps it puts us *on top* of the block without further ado. The bigger the block, the better the overall view! It is also important to *remain serene and open* in this process. If things don't work out at first, then something better is certainly waiting. Things have sometimes been taken away from under my nose, but what came afterward has always been better. Sometimes a solution will result that didn't look all that great at first; it only proves to be the optimal one in retrospect.

No matter how bleak the present may seem to be, *enjoy the little beauties of daily life*. Inside of each of us there is a master of the art of living who knows how to make the best of everything and make the little joys into major events. This master of the art of living also lets us pamper ourselves. When we become experts at this, we can also make the surrounding world happier with this art.

It is also important to know that everything that may develop – whether confidence, serenity, persistence, or humour – needs time, is related to setbacks, and exists more sometimes and less at others. Some people may use this book for a while, but lay it aside while the mudras work. Soon old patterns show up again. This isn't a problem since we can go back to the book and practise the mudras more frequently. Even though it may appear that we are once again completely at the beginning, this isn't the case. We will see the book with different eyes and experience new depths in the book and within ourselves. Our path is like a spiral that snakes around the mountain to the peak. Over and over, we pass the same side of the mountain where the path is difficult, but always on a higher level. So we must continue with open eyes and a happy mood.

Always stay in *a state of cheerful expectation*. What will we encounter around the next bend? What do we expect? No one can imagine all the awful things I thought would happen to me either sooner or later during the years before I practised yoga. My fantasy was boundless. We can either imagine everything that is wonderful – that makes us happy – or every illness, deepest loneliness, impoverishment, etc. Why not expect the best and then confidently see what comes? I have learned, and am still learning, to refine this ability. Try it, and then a new small or great adventure will be waiting behind every bend in the road. Time and time again I experience that my expectations are fulfiled. This is a cosmic law.

In short, practise the mudras in silence, and remain persistent and mindful while doing them. Always seek new solutions and remain open for something new. Always expect the best, and be happy about what is waiting. I will keep my fingers crossed for all of you!

BIBLIOGRAPHY

Bach, Edward. *Blumen, die durch die Seele heilen*. München, 1984; English
language readers may want to read *The Bach Flower Remedies*.
New Cannan, CT: Keats, 1997.

Berendt, Joachim-Ernst. *Ich höre – also bin ich*. München, 1993; English
language readers may want to read *The Third Ear: On Listening to
the World*. New York: Henry Holt & Co., 1995.

Berufsverband deutscher Yogalehrer (BDY). *Der Weg des Yoga*. Petersberg,
1991.

Braem, Harald. *Die Macht der Farben*. München, 1987.

Brooke, Elisabeth. *Von Salbei, Klee und Löwenzahn*. Freiburg, 1996.

Conrad, Jo and Benjamin Seiler. "Atmen Sie Sich gesund" in *ZeitenSchrift*,
5/95.

Da Silva, Kim. *Gesundheit in unseren Händen*. München, 1991.

———. *Richtig essen zur richtigen Zeit*. München, 1990.

Da Silva, Kim and Do-Ri Rydl. *Energie durch Bewegung*. Wien, 1997.

Eckert, Achim. *Das heilende Tao*. Frieburg, 1996.

Eggetsberger, Gerhard. *Charisma-Training*. Wien, 1993.

———. *Kopftraining der Sieger*. Wien, 1996.

———. *Power für den ganzen Tag*. Wien, 1995.

Felder, Pauline. *Gesundheits-Brevier*. Solothurn, 1993.

Friebe, Margarete. *Das Alpha-Training*. München, 1983.

Gach, Michael Reed. *Heilende Punkte*. München, 1992.

Goleman, Daniel. *Emotional Intelligence*. New York: Bantam, 1997.

Hesse, Herman. *Traumgeschenk*.

Hirschi, Gertrud. *Basic Yoga for Everybody*. York Beach, ME: Samuel Weiser, 1999.

————. *Innere Kräfte entdecken und nutzen*. Freiburg, 1996.

————. *Yoga für Seele, Geist und Körper*. Freiburg, 1993.

Höting, Hans. *Qi-Gong-Kugeln*. München, 1995

Hürlimann, Gertrud I. *Handlesen*. St. Gallen: Wettswil, 1996.

Johari, Harish. *Das große Chakra-Buch*. Frieburg, 1979; English language readers may want to read *Chakras: Energy Centers of Transformation*. Rochester, VT: Inner Traditions, 1987.

Lad, Vasant. *Ayurveda, the Science of Self-Healing: A Practical Guide*. Twin Lakes, WI: Lotus Light, 1990.

Lütge, Lothar-Rüdiger. *Kundalini: Die Erweckung der Lebenskraft*. Freiburg, 1989.

Mala, Matthias. *Handenergie*. München, 1993.

————. *Heilkraft der Sonnen-Meditation*. München, 1995.

————. *Magische Hände*. München: Hugendubel, 1998.

————. *Seelen-Energie deiner Fingeraura*. München, 1993.

Middendorf, Ilse. *Der erfahrbare Atem*. Paderborn, 1985.

Namikoshi, Tokujiro. *Japanese Finger Therapy*. New York: Japan Publications, 1994.

Ornish, Dean. *Dr. Dean Ornish's Program for Reversing Heart Disease*. New York: Random House, 1990.

Ramm-Bonwitt, Ingrid. *Mudras—Geheimsprache der Yogis*. Freiburg, 1988.

Rappenecker, Wilfried. *Fünf Elemente und Zwölf Meridiane*. Waldeck, 1996.

Reid, Lori. *Health in Your Hands: How to Gain a Detailed Picture of Your State of Health from Your Hands*. London: Aquarian Press, 1993.

Rodelli, Sofie. *Händeübungen als Heilgymnastik*. München 1961.

Ros, Frank. *The Lost Secrets of Ayurvedic Acupuncture: An Ayurvedic Guide to Acupuncture*. Twin Lakes, WI: Lotus Press, 1994.

Rueger, Christoph. *Die musikalische Hausapotheke*. München, 1991.

Sacharow, Boris. *Das große Geheimnis*. München, 1954.

Schiegl, Heinz. *Color-Therapie – Heilung durch Farbkraft*. Freiburg, 1982.

Schleberger, Eckart: *Die indische Götterwelt*. Köln, 1986.

Schrott, Ernst. *Gesund und jung mit Ayurveda*. München, 1996.

Schwarz, A. A., R. P. Schweppe, and W. M. Pfau. *Wyda – die Kraft der Druiden*. Freiburg, 1989.

Singh, Satya. *Das Kundalini Yoga Handbuch*. München, 1990.

Sriram, Angelika. *Lotosblüten öffnen sich: Indischer Tempeltanz*. München, 1989.

Storl, Wolf-Dieter. *Heilkräuter und Zauberpflanzen zwischen Haustür und Gartentor*. Aarau, 1996.

Swami Sivananda Radha. *Kundalini Praxis: Verbindung mit dem inneren Selbst*. Freiburg, 1992.

Swami Sayananda Saraswati. *Asana—Pranayama—Mudra—Bandha*. Hergensweiler, 1989.

Tawm, Kim. *Geheime Übungen taoistischer Mönche*. Frieburg, 1982.

Thyler, Maya. *Wohltuende Wickel*. Worb, 1993.

Wagner, Franz. *Akupressur leicht gemacht*. München, 1985.

Weber, Divo Helche. *Alta-Major Energie*. München, 1987.

INDEX

ABOUT THE AUTHOR

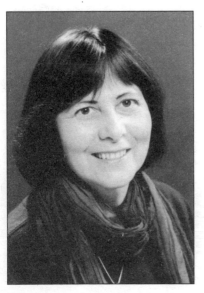

For the past 16 years, Gertrud Hirschi has taught yoga in accordance with the latest medical findings at her own yoga school in Zurich, Switzerland. She holds seminars in Switzerland, Germany, and Greece. She is also the author of *Basic Yoga for Everybody,* a book and card set, also published by Weiser.